Skills Performance Checklists

to accompany

FUNDAMENTAL NURSING

Concepts and Skills

SECOND EDITION

Grace Cole, RN

Coordinator/Instructor
Department of Vocational Nursing
Grayson County College
Denison, Texas

■ INTRODUCTION TO STUDENTS ■

The checklists in this book were developed to assist your instructors in evaluating your competence in performing the nursing interventions presented in the text *Fundamental Nursing Concepts and Skills*. Instructors can check "Satisfactory," "Unsatisfactory," or "Needs Practice" for each step. Specific instructions or feedback can be provided in the "Comments" column. These checklists are perforated so that you can easily remove them and turn them in as required. They have been streamlined to include *only* the critical steps needed to satisfactorily master the skill. They are *not* intended to replace the text that describes and illustrates in detail each nursing skill.

■ CONTENTS ■

**Performance Checklist
Skill 6–1**

PATIENT TEACHING

		S	U	Comments
1.	Assessed knowledge of material to be taught.	___	___	_____
2.	Assessed knowledge of patient illness or condition, including health promotion and coping with impaired function.	___	___	_____
3.	Decided what information or skill needs to be taught.	___	___	_____
4.	Assessed patient readiness and ability to learn, acceptance of illness or condition, language, and visual and hearing acuity.	___	___	_____
5.	Referred to medical record, care plan, or Kardex for special interventions.	___	___	_____
6.	Obtained equipment.	___	___	_____
7.	Introduced self.	___	___	_____
8.	Identified patient by identification band.	___	___	_____
9.	Explained procedure to be taught.	___	___	_____
10.	Washed hands and donned clean gloves according to agency policy, OSHA, and CDC guidelines.	___	___	_____
11.	Prepared patient for intervention.	___	___	_____
12.	Raised bed to comfortable working level.	___	___	_____
13.	Arranged for patient privacy.	___	___	_____
14.	Implemented teaching plan.	___	___	_____
15.	Praised efforts and success of patient.	___	___	_____
16.	Ended session with patient review of what was learned.	___	___	_____
17.	Removed gloves and washed hands.			
18.	Documented.	___	___	_____

Performance Checklist
Skill 7–1

ADMITTING A PATIENT

		S	U	Comments
1.	Checked assigned room, opened bed at appropriate height, and turned on light.	___	___	_____
2.	Obtained equipment.	___	___	_____
3.	Referred to medical record, care plan, or Kardex for special interventions.	___	___	_____
4.	Introduced self.	___	___	_____
5.	Identified patient by identification band.	___	___	_____
6.	Explained procedure to patient.	___	___	_____
7.	Washed hands and applied clean gloves.	___	___	_____
8.	Oriented patient to unit, lounge, and nurses' station if condition warranted.	___	___	_____
9.	Oriented patient to room and bathroom and taught use of equipment such as call system, bed, telephone, and television.	___	___	_____
10.	Prepared patient for intervention.	___	___	_____
11.	Raised bed to comfortable working level.	___	___	_____
12.	Arranged for patient privacy.	___	___	_____
13.	Assisted patient to undress if needed.	___	___	_____
14.	Followed agency policy for care of valuables, clothing, and medications.	___	___	_____
15.	Obtained patient's health history and performed initial nursing assessment.	___	___	_____
16.	Provided for safety with bed in low position and side rails up.	___	___	_____
17.	Reviewed preadmission test results.	___	___	_____
18.	Began nursing care.	___	___	_____
19.	Invited family back to room if they left earlier.	___	___	_____
20.	Explained diagnostic studies and nursing care to be administered.	___	___	_____
21.	Removed gloves and washed hands.	___	___	_____
22.	Documented.	___	___	_____

Performance Checklist
Skill 7–2

TRANSFERRING A PATIENT

	S	U	Comments

Intraagency Transfer

1. Obtained equipment.

2. Referred to medical record, care plan, or Kardex for special interventions.

3. Introduced self.

4. Identified patient by identification band.

5. Explained procedure to patient.

6. Washed hands and donned clean gloves.

7. Gathered patient's belongings and necessary care items, health records, and medications.

8. Prepared patient for intervention.

9. Raised bed to comfortable working level.

10. Arranged for patient privacy.

11. Assisted in transferring patient and monitored condition.

12. Gave personal belongings to nurse on receiving unit.

13. Deposited medical record and medications at nurses' station.

14. Introduced patient/family to nurses on new unit and assisted to bed.

15. Explained treatment, policies, and procedures that were different in new unit.

16. Notified other departments such as x-ray, laboratory, switchboard, dietary, and business office of transfer and new room number.

Interagency Transfer

17. Completed an interagency referral form and telephoned receiving agency to answer questions.

	S	U	Comments
18. Performed discharge procedure.	___	___	_____
19. Telephoned receiving agency that patient was being transported. Gave nurse a report on patient.	___	___	_____
20. Sent copy of medical record.	___	___	_____
21. Assisted patient to transporting vehicle by wheelchair or stretcher and assessed condition.	___	___	_____
22. Removed gloves and washed hands.	___	___	_____
23. Documented.	___	___	_____

**Performance Checklist
Skill 7–3**

DISCHARGING A PATIENT

		S	**U**	**Comments**
1.	Obtained equipment.	___	___	_____
2.	Referred to medical record, care plan, or Kardex for special interventions.	___	___	_____
3.	Introduced self.	___	___	_____
4.	Identified patient by identification band.	___	___	_____
5.	Explained procedure to patient.	___	___	_____
6.	Washed hands and donned clean gloves.	___	___	_____
7.	Prepared patient for intervention.	___	___	_____
8.	Raised bed to comfortable working level.	___	___	_____
9.	Arranged for patient privacy.	___	___	_____
10.	Verified verbally that patient understands home care instructions.	___	___	_____
11.	Assessed whether business office had released patient for discharge.	___	___	_____
12.	Checked clothing and valuable list according to agency policy.	___	___	_____
13.	Assisted patient to dress and pack belongings.	___	___	_____
14.	Assisted patient to wheelchair and escorted to waiting vehicle and assisted into vehicle.	___	___	_____
15.	Removed gloves and washed hands.	___	___	_____
16.	Documented.	___	___	_____

**Performance Checklist
Skill 10–1**

CARING FOR THE PATIENT WHO IS DYING

	S	U	Comments
1. Obtained equipment.	___	___	_____
2. Referred to medical record, care plan, or Kardex for special interventions.	___	___	_____
3. Introduced self.	___	___	_____
4. Identified patient by identification band.	___	___	_____
5. Explained procedure to patient.	___	___	_____
6. Washed hands and donned clean gloves.	___	___	_____
7. Prepared patient for intervention.	___	___	_____
8. Raised bed to comfortable working level.	___	___	_____
9. Arranged for patient privacy.	___	___	_____
10. Assessed patient needs.	___	___	_____
11. Provided comfort measures.	___	___	_____
12. Assessed for signs and symptoms of approaching death.	___	___	_____
13. Provided relief of pain.	___	___	_____
14. Allowed family members to assist in patient care when feasible.	___	___	_____
15. Assessed spiritual needs.	___	___	_____
16. Listened to patient and assessed affect.	___	___	_____
17. Talked honestly to patient, yet avoided telling anything physician had not shared.	___	___	_____
18. Explained to family about signs where applicable.	___	___	_____
19. Removed gloves and washed hands.	___	___	_____
20. Documented.	___	___	_____

Performance Checklist
Skill 10–2

ASSESSING THE TIME OF THE PATIENT'S DEATH

		S	U	Comments
1.	Obtained equipment.	___	___	_____
2.	Referred to medical record, care plan, or Kardex for special interventions.	___	___	_____
3.	Introduced self.	___	___	_____
4.	Identified patient by identification band.	___	___	_____
5.	Explained procedure to patient.	___	___	_____
6.	Washed hands and donned clean gloves.	___	___	_____
7.	Prepared patient for intervention.	___	___	_____
8.	Raised bed to comfortable working level.	___	___	_____
9.	Arranged for patient privacy.	___	___	_____
10.	Initiated CPR, if appropriate.	___	___	_____
11.	Assessed cessation of pulse, respiration, and blood pressure, and reported findings.	___	___	_____
12.	Notified attending physician.	___	___	_____
13.	Remained in room until physician arrived and made pronouncement of death.	___	___	_____
14.	Allowed family members to express their feelings.	___	___	_____
15.	Listened to family members and assessed their responses.	___	___	_____
16.	Removed gloves and washed hands.	___	___	_____
17.	Documented.	___	___	_____

**Performance Checklist
Skill 10–3**

CARING FOR THE BODY AFTER DEATH

		S	U	Comments
1.	Obtained equipment.	___	___	_____
2.	Referred to medical record, care plan, or Kardex for special interventions.	___	___	_____
3.	Washed hands and donned clean gloves.	___	___	_____
4.	Prepared deceased for intervention.	___	___	_____
5.	Raised bed to comfortable working level.			
6.	Arranged for privacy and prevented other patients from seeing into room.	___	___	_____
7.	Explained to family regarding nursing activity and asked to leave room unless religious beliefs necessitate their assistance with body.	___	___	_____
8.	Closed patient's eyes and mouth if necessary.	___	___	_____
9.	Removed all tubes and other devices from patient's body.	___	___	_____
10.	Placed patient in supine position.	___	___	_____
11.	Replaced soiled dressing with clean ones.	___	___	_____
12.	Bathed patient as necessary.	___	___	_____
13.	Brushed or combed hair.	___	___	_____
14.	Applied clean gown.	___	___	_____
15.	Cared for valuables and personal belongings and documented dispersement.	___	___	_____
16.	Allowed family to view patient and remained in room.	___	___	_____
17.	Attached special label if patient had contagious disease.	___	___	_____
18.	Awaited arrival of ambulance or transferred to morgue or followed agency policy.	___	___	_____
19.	Removed gloves and washed hands.	___	___	_____
20.	Documented.	___	___	_____

Performance Checklist
Skill 11–1

MEASURING BODY TEMPERATURE (ORAL, AXILLARY, RECTAL)

	S	U	Comments
1. Obtained equipment.	___	___	_____
2. Referred to medical record, care plan, or Kardex for special interventions.	___	___	_____
3. Introduced self.	___	___	_____
4. Identified patient by identification band.	___	___	_____
5. Explained procedure to patient.	___	___	_____
6. Washed hands and donned clean gloves.	___	___	_____
7. Prepared patient for intervention.	___	___	_____
8. Raised bed to comfortable working level.	___	___	_____
9. Arranged for patient privacy.	___	___	_____

Oral temperature with glass thermometer

	S	U	Comments
10. Removed clinical thermometer from container, being careful not to touch tip of thermometer.	___	___	_____
11. Held thermometer at eye level, rotated until mercury line was visible, and read.	___	___	_____
12. Shook thermometer down to 96° F or 35.5° C using a snapping motion of wrist while holding tip end of thermometer firmly between thumb and first two forefingers.	___	___	_____
13. Applied plastic sheath to thermometer.	___	___	_____
14. Placed thermometer tip gently under tongue to side, midline (R. or L. of sublingual pocket).	___	___	_____
15. Instructed patient to hold thermometer in mouth and to keep lips closed.	___	___	_____
16. Kept thermometer in place at least 2 or 3 minutes or according to agency policy.	___	___	_____
17. Removed plastic sheath and discarded.	___	___	_____
18. Held thermometer horizontally at eye level and read to one tenth degree accuracy.	___	___	_____

	S	**U**	**Comments**

19. Shook thermometer down.

20. Returned thermometer to container.

21. Made patient comfortable.

22. Removed gloves and washed hands.

23. Documented.

Rectal temperature with glass thermometer

24. Placed patient in left side-lying position.

25. Applied plastic sheath over a stubby or pear-shaped thermometer tip.

26. Lubricated bulb end of thermometer with water-soluble lubricant. For adult: lubricated 1 to 1.5 inches. For infant or young child: lubricated about 0.5 to 1 inch.

27. Exposed only rectal area, separated cheeks of buttocks, and visualized anus.

28. Asked patient to take a deep breath.

29. Inserted thermometer gently into rectum.

30. Permitted buttocks to fall in place and held thermometer in place for 3 to 5 minutes or according to agency policy.

31. Removed rectal thermometer gently, peeled off plastic sheath, and discarded.

32. Cleaned rectal area if necessary.

33. Held thermometer horizontally at eye level and read to one tenth degree accuracy.

34. Shook thermometer down.

35. Returned thermometer to container.

36. Made patient comfortable.

37. Removed gloves and washed hands.

38. Documented.

Axillary temperature with glass thermometer

39. Placed patient in supine position.

40. Applied plastic sheath over oral thermometer tip.

41. Placed oral thermometer into center of axilla, lowered patient's arm over thermometer, and placed patient's arm across chest.

42. Held thermometer in place for 5 to 10 minutes or according to agency policy.

43. Removed thermometer carefully.

Performance Check List
Skill 11–1

MEASURING BODY TEMPERATURE
(ORAL, AXILLARY, RECTAL) (Continued)

		S	U	Comments
44.	Held thermometer horizontally at eye level and read to one tenth degree accuracy.	____	____	_____
45.	Shook thermometer down.	____	____	_____
46.	Returned thermometer to container.	____	____	_____
47.	Made patient comfortable.	____	____	_____
48.	Removed gloves and washed hands.	____	____	_____
49.	Documented	____	____	_____

Performance Checklist
Skill 11–2

MEASURING PULSE (RADIAL, APICAL)

		S	U	Comments
1.	Obtained equipment.	___	___	_____
2.	Referred to medical record, care plan, or Kardex for special interventions.	___	___	_____
3.	Introduced self.	___	___	_____
4.	Identified patient by identification band.	___	___	_____
5.	Explained procedure to patient.	___	___	_____
6.	Washed hands and donned clean gloves.	___	___	_____
7.	Prepared patient for intervention.	___	___	_____
8.	Raised bed to comfortable working level.	___	___	_____
9.	Arranged for patient privacy.	___	___	_____

Radial Pulse

		S	U	Comments
10.	Positioned patient's arm for comfort and for easy access for nurse.	___	___	_____
11.	Placed first three fingers of dominant hand over and parallel to radial artery and lightly compressed against the radius.	___	___	_____
12.	Counted number of pulsations for 1 minute.	___	___	_____
13.	Noted rate, rhythm, and strength of pulse.	___	___	_____
14.	Removed gloves and washed hands.	___	___	_____
15.	Documented.	___	___	_____

Apical Pulse

		S	U	Comments
16.	Positioned patient on back.	___	___	_____
17.	Moved patient gown to make upper chest visible without exposing patient.	___	___	_____
18.	Palpated fifth intercostal space and moved to left midclavicular line.	___	___	_____
19.	Placed diaphragm of stethoscope on apex of heart and listened for "lub dub" sounds (beats).	___	___	_____

	S	U	Comments
20. Counted number of heart beats for 1 minute.	____	____	_____
21. Noted rate, rhythm, and strength of pulse.	____	____	_____
22. Made patient comfortable.	____	____	_____
23. Removed gloves and washed hands.	____	____	_____
24. Documented.	____	____	_____

**Performance Checklist
Skill 11–3**

MEASURING RESPIRATIONS

	S	U	Comments
1. Referred to medical record, care plan, or Kardex for special interventions.	___	___	_____
2. Introduced self.	___	___	_____
3. Identified patient by identification band.	___	___	_____
4. Explained procedure to patient.	___	___	_____
5. Washed hands and donned clean gloves.	___	___	_____
6. Prepared patient for intervention.	___	___	_____
7. Raised bed to comfortable working level.	___	___	_____
8. Arranged for patient privacy.	___	___	_____
9. Kept fingers in place after counting the pulse.	___	___	_____
10. Counted the rise and fall of patient's chest for 1 minute.	___	___	_____
11. If unable to easily see breathing, moved patient's arm across abdomen or lower chest or placed own hand on patient's shoulder.	___	___	_____
12. While counting respirations, assessed rate, depth, and rhythm.	___	___	_____
13. Made patient comfortable.	___	___	_____
14. Removed gloves and washed hands.	___	___	_____
15. Documented.	___	___	_____

Performance Checklist
Skill 11–4

MEASURING BLOOD PRESSURE

		S	U	Comments
1.	Obtained equipment.	___	___	_____
2.	Referred to medical record, care plan, or Kardex for special interventions.	___	___	_____
3.	Introduced self.	___	___	_____
4.	Identified patient by identification band.	___	___	_____
5.	Explained procedure to patient.	___	___	_____
6.	Washed hands and donned clean gloves.	___	___	_____
7.	Prepared patient for intervention.	___	___	_____
8.	Raised bed to comfortable working level.	___	___	_____
9.	Arranged for patient privacy.	___	___	_____
10.	Exposed upper arm fully.	___	___	_____
11.	Palpated brachial artery in antecubital space.	___	___	_____
12.	Located middle of inflatable bladder and positioned middle of lower edge of cuff 1 inch above brachial artery pulsation.	___	___	_____
13.	Made certain cuff was fully deflated and wrapped it evenly and snugly around arm.	___	___	_____
14.	Positioned manometer at eye level.	___	___	_____
15.	Tightened screw valve but not too tight.	___	___	_____
16.	Placed diaphragm of stethoscope over brachial artery.	___	___	_____
17.	Placed stethoscope earpieces in ears.	___	___	_____
18.	Inflated cuff to 160 to 180.	___	___	_____
19.	Released valve slowly, allowing mercury to fall at a rate of two to three points per second.	___	___	_____
20.	Noted point on manometer at which first sound is heard and read pressure to nearest even number.	___	___	_____

	S	U	Comments

21. Continued to deflate cuff gradually and noted point at which a muffled sound appears. _____ _____ _____

22. Continued to slowly deflate cuff and noted point at which last number is heard. _____ _____ _____

23. Completed deflation rapidly and removed cuff from arm. _____ _____ _____

24. If need to retake blood pressure, waited at least 30 seconds before repeating procedure. _____ _____ _____

25. Removed, folded, and stored cuff and cleaned earpieces of stethoscope. _____ _____ _____

26. Made patient comfortable. _____ _____ _____

27. Removed gloves and washed hands. _____ _____ _____

28. Documented. _____ _____ _____

Performance Checklist
Skill 12–1

PERFORMING A GENERAL SURVEY

	S	U	Comments
1. Obtained equipment.	___	___	_____
2. Referred to medical record, care plan, or Kardex for special interventions.	___	___	_____
3. Introduced self.	___	___	_____
4. Identified patient by identification band.	___	___	_____
5. Explained procedure to patient.	___	___	_____
6. Washed hands and donned clean gloves.	___	___	_____
7. Prepared patient for intervention.	___	___	_____
8. Raised bed to comfortable working level.	___	___	_____
9. Arranged for patient privacy.	___	___	_____
10. Reviewed patient's health history.	___	___	_____
11. Assessed patient clinically, such as behavior, color, hair color and texture, emotional state, overall looks versus stated age, and general look of health.	___	___	_____
12. Included assessment of sex, ethnic origin, signs of distress or severe pain, posture, body type or build, gait, cleanliness, grooming, odor, speech, and possible patient abuse.	___	___	_____
13. Removed gloves and washed hands.	___	___	_____
14. Documented.	___	___	_____

Performance Checklist
Skill 12–2

ASSESSING THE SKIN

	S	U	Comments
1. Obtained equipment.			
2. Referred to medical record, care plan, or Kardex for special interventions.			
3. Introduced self.			
4. Identified patient by identification band.			
5. Explained procedure to patient.			
6. Washed hands and donned clean gloves.			
7. Prepared patient for intervention.			
8. Raised bed to comfortable working level.			
9. Arranged for patient privacy.			
10. Inspected skin surfaces for color and presence of lesions; compared opposite body parts.			
11. Inspected color of lips, oral mucous membranes, nail beds, sclerae, conjunctivae, and palms of hands.			
12. Palpated skin surfaces with fingers to determine moisture and texture of skin; assessed secretions.			
13. Tested for skin turgor; when skin was released, noted how long it took to return to normal position.			
14. Assessed temperature of skin by using back of hand; compared opposite sides of body.			
15. If lesions were detected, noted size, color, location, and type; palpated gently to determine shape, mobility, and character; asked patient whether there was any pain or tenderness during palpation.			
16. Assessed for edema by inspecting feet, ankles, sacral area, and scapular areas; assessed degree of edema by pressing with thumb for 5 seconds.			
17. Removed gloves and washed hands.			
18. Documented.			

**Performance Checklist
Skill 12–3**

ASSESSING THE HAIR AND SCALP

	S	U	Comments
1. Obtained equipment.	___	___	_____
2. Referred to medical record, care plan, or Kardex for special interventions.	___	___	_____
3. Introduced self.	___	___	_____
4. Identified patient by identification band.	___	___	_____
5. Explained procedure to patient.	___	___	_____
6. Washed hands and donned clean gloves.	___	___	_____
7. Prepared patient for intervention.	___	___	_____
8. Raised bed to comfortable working level.	___	___	_____
9. Arranged for patient privacy.	___	___	_____
10. Inspected hair for color, thickness, distribution, and texture.	___	___	_____
11. Inspected hair shaft and follicles to determine presence of lice.	___	___	_____
12. Inspected scalp for cleanliness and lesions by separating hair.	___	___	_____
13. Inspected hair for distribution over lower extremities.	___	___	_____
14. Removed gloves and washed hands.	___	___	_____
15. Documented.	___	___	_____

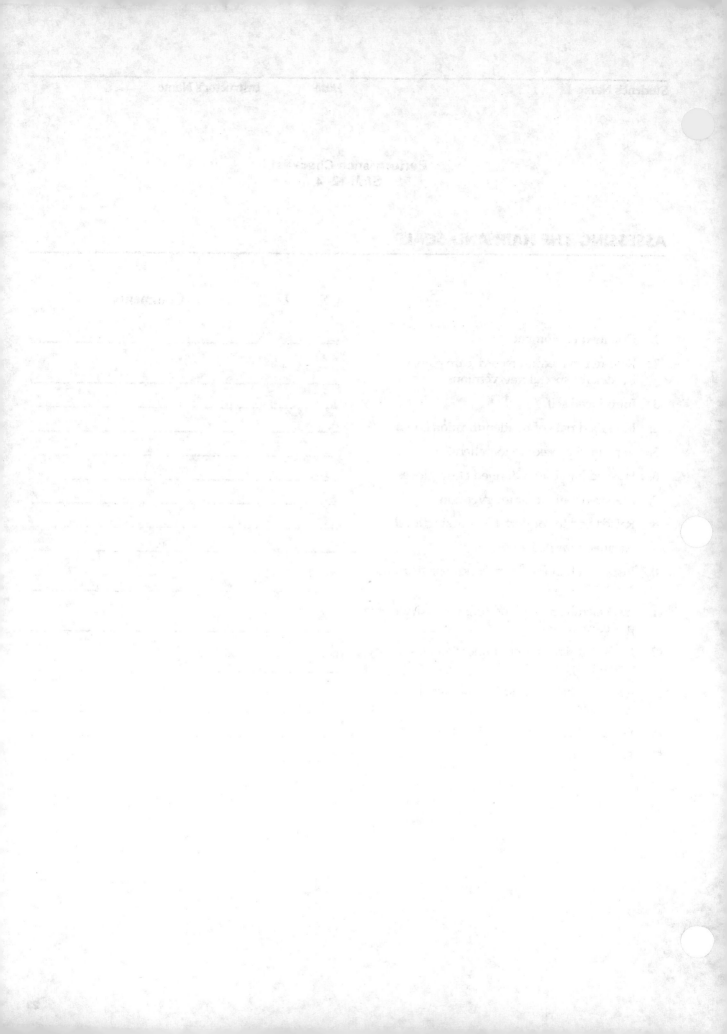

**Performance Checklist
Skill 12–4**

ASSESSING THE NAILS

		S	U	Comments
1.	Obtained equipment.	____	____	_____
2.	Referred to medical record, care plan, or Kardex for special interventions.	____	____	_____
3.	Introduced self.	____	____	_____
4.	Identified patient by identification band.	____	____	_____
5.	Explained procedure to patient.	____	____	_____
6.	Washed hands and donned clean gloves.	____	____	_____
7.	Prepared patient for intervention.	____	____	_____
8.	Raised bed to comfortable working level.	____	____	_____
9.	Arranged for patient privacy.	____	____	_____
10.	Inspected nails for color, thickness, shape, and curvature.	____	____	_____
11.	Assessed capillary refill by applying pressure with thumb to patient's nail beds.	____	____	_____
12.	Removed gloves and washed hands.	____	____	_____
13.	Documented.	____	____	_____

**Performance Checklist
Skill 12–5**

ASSESSING THE EYES

		S	U	Comments
1.	Obtained equipment.	____	____	_____
2.	Referred to medical record, care plan, or Kardex for special interventions.	____	____	_____
3.	Introduced self.	____	____	_____
4.	Identified patient by identification band.	____	____	_____
5.	Explained procedure to patient.	____	____	_____
6.	Washed hands and donned clean gloves.	____	____	_____
7.	Prepared patient for intervention.	____	____	_____
8.	Raised bed to comfortable working level.	____	____	_____
9.	Arranged for patient privacy.	____	____	_____
10.	Inspected external eye structures.	____	____	_____
11.	Examined eyes for position and alignment.	____	____	_____
12.	Inspected eyebrows for position, hair growth, and movement.	____	____	_____
13.	Inspected eyelids for position.	____	____	_____
14.	Inspected eyelids and sclerae for color, edema, inflammation, and lesions.	____	____	_____
15.	Looked for excess tears, signs of inflammation, infection, edema, and tumors and looked at underside of eyelids.	____	____	_____
16.	Assessed pupils for size and shape and tested pupillary response.	____	____	_____
17.	Removed gloves and washed hands.	____	____	_____
18.	Documented.	____	____	_____

Performance Checklist
Skill 12–6

ASSESSING THE EARS

		S	U	Comments
1.	Obtained equipment.	____	____	_____
2.	Referred to medical record, care plan, or Kardex for special interventions.	____	____	_____
3.	Introduced self.	____	____	_____
4.	Identified patient by identification band.	____	____	_____
5.	Explained procedure to patient.	____	____	_____
6.	Washed hands and donned clean gloves.	____	____	_____
7.	Prepared patient for intervention.	____	____	_____
8.	Raised bed to comfortable working level.	____	____	_____
9.	Arranged for patient privacy.	____	____	_____
10.	Inspected opening of ear canal.	____	____	_____
11.	Assessed patient's hearing acuity.	____	____	_____
12.	Used a tuning fork if more precise assessment of hearing was needed.	____	____	_____
13.	Performed Weber's test if needed.	____	____	_____
14.	Performed Rhine test if needed.	____	____	_____
15.	Used otoscope to examine ear canals.	____	____	_____
16.	Removed gloves and washed hands.	____	____	_____
17.	Documented.	____	____	_____

**Performance Checklist
Skill 12–7**

ASSESSING THE NOSE AND SINUSES

	S	U	Comments
1. Obtained equipment.	___	___	_____
2. Referred to medical record, care plan, or Kardex for special interventions.	___	___	_____
3. Introduced self.	___	___	_____
4. Identified patient by identification band.	___	___	_____
5. Explained procedure to patient.	___	___	_____
6. Washed hands and donned clean gloves.	___	___	_____
7. Prepared patient for intervention.	___	___	_____
8. Raised bed to comfortable working level.	___	___	_____
9. Arranged for patient privacy.	___	___	_____
10. Inspected nose.	___	___	_____
11. Inspected mucosa using penlight.	___	___	_____
12. Inspected inner nares using speculum.	___	___	_____
13. Examined frontal and maxillary sinuses.	___	___	_____
14. Removed gloves and washed hands.	___	___	_____
15. Documented.	___	___	_____

Performance Checklist
Skill 12–8

ASSESSING THE MOUTH AND PHARYNX

		S	U	Comments
1.	Obtained equipment.	___	___	_____
2.	Referred to medical record, care plan, or Kardex for special interventions.	___	___	_____
3.	Introduced self.	___	___	_____
4.	Identified patient by identification band.	___	___	_____
5.	Explained procedure to patient.	___	___	_____
6.	Washed hands and donned clean gloves.	___	___	_____
7.	Prepared patient for intervention.	___	___	_____
8.	Raised bed to comfortable working level.	___	___	_____
9.	Arranged for patient privacy.	___	___	_____
10.	Inspected lips.	___	___	_____
11.	Asked patient to open mouth slightly and examined oral mucosa.	___	___	_____
12.	Inspected buccal mucosa using penlight.	___	___	_____
13.	Inspected patient's gums using tongue depressor.	___	___	_____
14.	Asked patient to open mouth wide and inspected all surfaces of teeth.	___	___	_____
15.	Removed gloves and washed hands.	___	___	_____
16.	Documented.	___	___	_____

Performance Checklist
Skill 12–9

ASSESSING THE STRUCTURES OF THE NECK

	S	U	Comments
1. Obtained equipment.	___	___	_____
2. Referred to medical record, care plan, or Kardex for special interventions.	___	___	_____
3. Introduced self.	___	___	_____
4. Identified patient by identification band.	___	___	_____
5. Explained procedure to patient.	___	___	_____
6. Washed hands and donned clean gloves.	___	___	_____
7. Prepared patient for intervention.	___	___	_____
8. Raised bed to comfortable working level.	___	___	_____
9. Arranged for patient privacy.	___	___	_____
10. Asked patient to move head and neck through full range of motion.	___	___	_____
11. Inspected neck for scars or masses.	___	___	_____
12. Palpated any masses felt to determine size, shape, and mobility.	___	___	_____
13. Palpated gently each side of neck and under chin using fingers of one hand to assess for lymph nodes.	___	___	_____
14. Palpated trachea using thumb and first finger of one hand.	___	___	_____
15. Palpated carotid pulse on each side of neck.	___	___	_____
16. Auscultated over carotid arteries for bruit.	___	___	_____
17. Removed gloves and washed hands.	___	___	_____
18. Documented.	___	___	_____

Performance Checklist
Skill 12–10

ASSESSING THE THORAX AND LUNGS

		S	U	Comments
1.	Obtained equipment.	___	___	_____
2.	Referred to medical record, care plan, or Kardex for special interventions.	___	___	_____
3.	Introduced self.	___	___	_____
4.	Identified patient by identification band.	___	___	_____
5.	Explained procedure to patient.	___	___	_____
6.	Washed hands and donned clean gloves.	___	___	_____
7.	Prepared patient for intervention.	___	___	_____
8.	Raised bed to comfortable working level.	___	___	_____
9.	Arranged for patient privacy.	___	___	_____
10.	Stood behind patient and inspected posterior thorax for shape, contour, posture, and deformities.	___	___	_____
11.	Palpated posterior chest wall to determine mass, areas of tenderness, and deformities.	___	___	_____
12.	Assessed for fremitus over intercostal spaces.	___	___	_____
13.	Percussed chest wall.	___	___	_____
14.	Listened to lung sounds.	___	___	_____
15.	Removed gloves and washed hands.	___	___	_____
16.	Documented.	___	___	_____

Performance Checklist
Skill 12–11

ASSESSING THE HEART AND VASCULAR SYSTEM

		S	U	Comments
1.	Obtained equipment.	___	___	_____
2.	Referred to medical record, care plan, or Kardex for special interventions.	___	___	_____
3.	Introduced self.	___	___	_____
4.	Identified patient by identification band.	___	___	_____
5.	Explained procedure to patient.	___	___	_____
6.	Washed hands and donned clean gloves.	___	___	_____
7.	Prepared patient for intervention.	___	___	_____
8.	Raised bed to comfortable working level.	___	___	_____
9.	Arranged for patient privacy.	___	___	_____
10.	Inspected neck and precordium for vein distention or pulsations.	___	___	_____
11.	Palpated chest over anatomic landmarks.	___	___	_____
12.	Auscultated heart sounds.	___	___	_____
13.	Identified first (S_1) and second (S_2) heart sounds.	___	___	_____
14.	Auscultated for extra sounds.	___	___	_____
15.	Auscultated apical pulse and counted beats for 1 minute.	___	___	_____
16.	Assessed pulses:			
	• Carotid pulse	___	___	_____
	• Radial pulse	___	___	_____
	• Brachial pulse	___	___	_____
	• Femoral pulse	___	___	_____
	• Popliteal pulse	___	___	_____
	• Dorsalis pulse	___	___	_____
	• Posterior tibial pulse	___	___	_____

	S	U	Comments

17. Sought assistance if pulses are not present; used an ultrasonic stethoscope.   ____ ____ _____

18. Removed gloves and washed hands.   ____ ____ _____

19. Documented.   ____ ____ _____

Performance Checklist
Skill 12–12

ASSESSING THE ABDOMEN

	S	U	Comments
1. Obtained equipment.	___	___	_____
2. Referred to medical record, care plan, or Kardex for special interventions.	___	___	_____
3. Introduced self.	___	___	_____
4. Identified patient by identification band.	___	___	_____
5. Explained procedure to patient.	___	___	_____
6. Washed hands and donned clean gloves.	___	___	_____
7. Prepared patient for intervention.	___	___	_____
8. Raised bed to comfortable working level.	___	___	_____
9. Arranged for patient privacy.	___	___	_____
10. Inspected abdomen for venous patterns, white striae on skin, and artificial openings.	___	___	_____
11. Assessed shape and symmetry, masses, or bulges of abdomen.	___	___	_____
12. Assessed for movement or pulsations of abdomen by looking across from side to side.	___	___	_____
13. Measured size of abdominal girth.	___	___	_____
14. Placed diaphragm of stethoscope and auscultated over each quadrant of abdomen.	___	___	_____
15. Auscultated for vascular sounds; notified physician of reported bruit.	___	___	_____
16. Palpated each abdominal quadrant; assessed for masses and areas of tenderness.	___	___	_____
17. Removed gloves and washed hands.	___	___	_____
18. Documented.	___	___	_____

**Performance Checklist
Skill 12–13**

ASSESSING THE BREASTS AND AXILLAE

		S	U	Comments
1.	Obtained equipment.	___	___	_____
2.	Referred to medical record, care plan, or Kardex for special interventions.	___	___	_____
3.	Introduced self.	___	___	_____
4.	Identified patient by identification band.	___	___	_____
5.	Explained procedure to patient.	___	___	_____
6.	Washed hands and donned clean gloves.	___	___	_____
7.	Prepared patient for intervention.	___	___	_____
8.	Raised bed to comfortable working level.	___	___	_____
9.	Arranged for patient privacy.	___	___	_____

Female patient

		S	U	Comments
10.	Inspected breasts for size, symmetry, shape, change in tissue, lumps, and contour.	___	___	_____
11.	Asked patient to place hands behind head or on hips and inspected breasts for flattening or unevenness.	___	___	_____
12.	Inspected skin for color, vascular markings, and puckering.	___	___	_____
13.	Inspected nipples and surrounding areola for shape, size and color, and discharge.	___	___	_____
14.	Placed patient in supine position with right hand under head and palpated right breast, pressing tissue against chest wall, one quadrant at a time; then moved in a clockwise direction, examining each quadrant.	___	___	_____
15.	Compressed nipple gently between thumb and finger to assess for discharge.	___	___	_____
16.	Palpated axillae gently and along inner aspect of upper arm to examine lymph nodes.	___	___	_____
17.	Repeated procedure for left breast.	___	___	_____

50

Male patient

18. Assessed nipples, areola, and breast tissue for welling, discharge, lumps, and lesions in same fashion as for female. _____ _____ _____

19. Removed gloves and washed hands. _____ _____ _____

20. Documented. _____ _____ _____

**Performance Checklist
Skill 12–14**

ASSESSING THE FEMALE GENITALIA AND RECTUM

	S	U	Comments
1. Obtained equipment.	___	___	_____
2. Referred to medical record, care plan, or Kardex for special interventions.	___	___	_____
3. Introduced self.	___	___	_____
4. Identified patient by identification band.	___	___	_____
5. Explained procedure to patient.	___	___	_____
6. Washed hands and donned clean gloves.	___	___	_____
7. Prepared patient for intervention.	___	___	_____
8. Raised bed to comfortable working level.	___	___	_____
9. Arranged for patient privacy.	___	___	_____

Vaginal examination

	S	U	Comments
10. Inspected external genitalia for distribution and thickness of pubic hair, color of skin, size and shape of labia, edema, and signs of infection.	___	___	_____
11. Separated labia and inspected clitoris and urinary meatus; assessed for inflammation, drainage, lesions, and masses.	___	___	_____
12. Examined vaginal opening, asked patient to bear down as if urinating, and assessed for bulging or protrusion through vaginal opening.	___	___	_____
13. Selected appropriate size speculum and warmed blades.	___	___	_____
14. Sat facing patient's perineum, inserted speculum into vagina at 45 degree angle, and locked speculum in open position once cervical os was visualized.	___	___	_____
15. Collected specimen for Pap smear and other smears if necessary.	___	___	_____
16. Inspected vaginal walls for color, presence of lesions, masses, drainage, and odor as speculum is closed and withdrawn.	___	___	_____

	S	U	Comments

Rectal examination

17. Inspected rectum for presence of external hemorrhoids, fissures, and other lesions. ____ ____ _____

18. Removed gloves, washed hands, and donned clean gloves; lubricated index finger. ____ ____ _____

19. Asked patient to bear down as if trying to have bowel movement. ____ ____ _____

20. Inserted index finger gently into rectum and angled toward patient's umbilicus; palpated walls of rectum for masses or nodules, asked patient if had pain or tenderness, and asked patient again to bear down and tighten sphincter muscle; removed finger from rectum. ____ ____ _____

21. Removed gloves and washed hands. ____ ____ _____

22. Documented. ____ ____ _____

**Performance Checklist
Skill 12–15**

ASSESSING THE MALE GENITALIA AND RECTUM

	S	U	Comments
1. Obtained equipment.	___	___	_____
2. Referred to medical record, care plan, or Kardex for special interventions.	___	___	_____
3. Introduced self.	___	___	_____
4. Identified patient by identification band.	___	___	_____
5. Explained procedure to patient.	___	___	_____
6. Washed hands and donned clean gloves.	___	___	_____
7. Prepared patient for intervention.	___	___	_____
8. Raised bed to comfortable working level.	___	___	_____
9. Arranged for patient privacy.	___	___	_____

Genitalia

	S	U	Comments
10. Inspected penis, assessing position of urethral opening, presence or absence of foreskin, color of skin, and presence of lesions, inflammation, and drainage.	___	___	_____
11. Inspected scrotum for symmetry, shape, skin color, and lesions.	___	___	_____
12. Assessed inguinal area palpating for lymph nodes, bulges, and hernias.	___	___	_____
13. Asked patient to lean forward and rest body on bed.	___	___	_____
14. Spread cheeks of buttocks and inspected anus for hemorrhoids or breaks in skin.	___	___	_____
15. Removed gloves and washed hands.	___	___	_____
16. Documented.	___	___	_____

Performance Checklist
Skill 12–16

ASSESSING THE MUSCULOSKELETAL SYSTEM

	S	U	Comments
1. Obtained equipment.	___	___	_____
2. Referred to medical record, care plan, or Kardex for special interventions.	___	___	_____
3. Introduced self.	___	___	_____
4. Identified patient by identification band.	___	___	_____
5. Explained procedure to patient.	___	___	_____
6. Washed hands and donned clean gloves.	___	___	_____
7. Prepared patient for intervention.	___	___	_____
8. Raised bed to comfortable working level.	___	___	_____
9. Arranged for patient privacy.	___	___	_____
10. Assessed patient walking and limping, deformity, or abnormalities of balance.	___	___	_____
11. Assessed patient's posture.	___	___	_____
12. Asked patient to move each joint through full range of motion.	___	___	_____
13. Assessed patient's muscle strength.	___	___	_____
14. Examined joints of upper and lower body, assessing for edema and inflammation; palpated for tenderness, malformation, nodules, and pain.	___	___	_____
15. Removed gloves and washed hands.	___	___	_____
16. Documented.	___	___	_____

Performance Checklist
Skill 12–17

ASSESSING THE NEUROLOGIC SYSTEM

	S	U	Comments
1. Obtained equipment.	___	___	_____
2. Referred to medical record, care plan, or Kardex for special interventions.	___	___	_____
3. Introduced self.	___	___	_____
4. Identified patient by identification band.	___	___	_____
5. Explained procedure to patient.	___	___	_____
6. Washed hands and donned clean gloves.	___	___	_____
7. Prepared patient for intervention.	___	___	_____
8. Raised bed to comfortable working level.	___	___	_____
9. Arranged for patient privacy.	___	___	_____
10. Assessed patient's level of consciousness.	___	___	_____
11. Asked questions such as "What is your name? Where are you? What day is this?"	___	___	_____
12. Gave commands for communication if patient unable to speak.	___	___	_____
13. Tested patient's response to painful stimuli.	___	___	_____
14. Assessed intellectual status and memory of past events.	___	___	_____
15. Assessed abstract ideas by asking meaning of phrases.	___	___	_____
16. Removed gloves and washed hands.	___	___	_____
17. Documented.	___	___	_____

Performance Checklist
Skill 13–1

MEASURING CAPILLARY BLOOD GLUCOSE LEVELS

		S	U	Comments
1.	Obtained equipment.			
2.	Referred to medical record, care plan, or Kardex for special interventions.			
3.	Introduced self.			
4.	Identified patient by identification band.			
5.	Explained procedure to patient.			
6.	Washed hands and donned clean gloves.			
7.	Prepared patient for intervention.			
8.	Raised bed to comfortable working level.			
9.	Arranged for patient privacy.			
10.	Removed cap from lancet using sterile technique.			
11.	Placed lancet into automatic lancing device according to instructions in operating manual.			
12.	Selected site on side of any fingertip; used heel for infant.			
13.	Wiped site with alcohol swab and discarded.			
14.	Asked patient to hold arm at side for 30 seconds.			
15.	Squeezed fingertip gently with thumb of same hand.			
16.	Held lancing device appropriately.			
17.	Placed trigger platform of lancing device on side of finger and pressed.			
18.	Squeezed finger in downward motion and wiped off first drop of blood.			
19.	Held strip level and touched drop of blood to test pad.			

	S	U	Comments

20. Began recommended timing; placed reagent strip into meter; after 60 seconds, blotted blood off test strip in appropriate site on meter and waited for numeric read out.

    ____ ____ _____

21. Removed lancet from device and discarded.

    ____ ____ _____

22. Removed gloves and washed hands.

    ____ ____ _____

23. Documented.

    ____ ____ _____

**Performance Checklist
Skill 13–2**

COLLECTING A MIDSTREAM URINE SPECIMEN

		S	U	Comments
1.	Obtained equipment.	____	____	_____
2.	Referred to medical record, care plan, or Kardex for special interventions.	____	____	_____
3.	Introduced self.	____	____	_____
4.	Identified patient by identification band.	____	____	_____
5.	Explained procedure to patient.	____	____	_____
6.	Washed hands and donned clean gloves.	____	____	_____
7.	Prepared patient for intervention.	____	____	_____
8.	Raised bed to comfortable working level.	____	____	_____
9.	Arranged for patient privacy.	____	____	_____
10.	Instructed patient to open midstream kit and cleanse perineum.	____	____	_____
11.	Requested patient to collect midstream specimen.	____	____	_____
12.	Secured lid on container.	____	____	_____
13.	Cleansed collector and returned to toilet seat, if applicable.	____	____	_____
14.	Labeled specimen.	____	____	_____
15.	Took urine specimen to laboratory with requisition in biohazard bag.	____	____	_____
16.	Removed gloves and washed hands.	____	____	_____
17.	Documented.	____	____	_____

Performance Checklist
Skill 13–3

COLLECTING A STERILE URINE SPECIMEN

	S	U	Comments
1. Obtained equipment.	___	___	_____
2. Referred to medical record, care plan, or Kardex for special interventions.	___	___	_____
3. Introduced self.	___	___	_____
4. Identified patient by identification band.	___	___	_____
5. Explained procedure to patient.	___	___	_____
6. Washed hands and donned clean gloves.	___	___	_____
7. Prepared patient for intervention.	___	___	_____
8. Raised bed to comfortable working level.	___	___	_____
9. Arranged for patient privacy.	___	___	_____

Catheter port collection

	S	U	Comments
10. Clamped just below catheter port for 30 minutes.	___	___	_____
11. Returned in 30 minutes and cleansed port with alcohol prep.	___	___	_____
12. Inserted needle into port at 30 degree angle and withdrew urine specimen.	___	___	_____
13. Placed urine in sterile specimen cup and unclamped catheter.	___	___	_____
14. Labeled specimen and took to laboratory with requisition.	___	___	_____

Straight catheter collection

	S	U	Comments
15. Opened catheter tray and prepared supplies using sterile technique.	___	___	_____
16. Placed sterile drape under patient's hips.	___	___	_____
17. Donned sterile gloves.	___	___	_____
18. Separated labia with thumb and index finger; using cotton ball, cleansed down from above clitoris to below anus and discarded wipe.	___	___	_____

	S	U	Comments

19. Lubricated catheter and inserted through urinary meatus. ____ ____ _____

20. When urine flowed, placed end of catheter in specimen cup and collected urine. ____ ____ _____

21. Placed lid on urine cup and labeled. Cleaned supplies. ____ ____ _____

22. Took urine specimen to laboratory with requisition using a biohazard bag. ____ ____ _____

23. Removed gloves and washed hands. ____ ____ _____

24. Documented. ____ ____ _____

Performance Checklist
Skill 13–4

COLLECTING A STOOL SPECIMEN

		S	U	Comments
1.	Obtained equipment.	___	___	_____
2.	Referred to medical record, care plan, or Kardex for special interventions.	___	___	_____
3.	Introduced self.	___	___	_____
4.	Identified patient by identification band.	___	___	_____
5.	Explained procedure to patient.	___	___	_____
6.	Washed hands and donned clean gloves.	___	___	_____
7.	Prepared patient for intervention.	___	___	_____
8.	Raised bed to comfortable working level.	___	___	_____
9.	Arranged for patient privacy.	___	___	_____
10.	Assisted patient to bathroom when necessary.	___	___	_____
11.	Requested patient to defecate into commode specimen device and prevented urine from entering specimen.	___	___	_____
12.	Transferred stool to specimen cup and closed lid.	___	___	_____
13.	Attached laboratory requisition and took to laboratory in a biohazard bag.	___	___	_____
14.	Removed gloves and washed hands.	___	___	_____
15.	Documented.	___	___	_____

Performance Checklist
Skill 13–5

MEASURING OCCULT BLOOD IN STOOL

	S	U	Comments
1. Obtained equipment.	___	___	_____
2. Referred to medical record, care plan, or Kardex for special interventions.	___	___	_____
3. Introduced self.	___	___	_____
4. Identified patient by identification band.	___	___	_____
5. Explained procedure to patient.	___	___	_____
6. Washed hands and donned clean gloves.	___	___	_____
7. Prepared patient for intervention.	___	___	_____
8. Raised bed to comfortable working level.	___	___	_____
9. Arranged for patient privacy.	___	___	_____
10. Collected stool specimen.	___	___	_____
11. Followed steps on Hemoccult slide test.	___	___	_____
12. Closed card and labeled.	___	___	_____
13. Took specimen to laboratory with requisition using a biohazard bag.	___	___	_____
14. Removed gloves and washed hands.	___	___	_____
15. Documented.	___	___	_____

Performance Checklist
Skill 13–6

COLLECTING SPUTUM

		S	U	Comments
1.	Obtained equipment.	___	___	_____
2.	Referred to medical record, care plan, or Kardex for special interventions.	___	___	_____
3.	Introduced self.	___	___	_____
4.	Identified patient by identification band.	___	___	_____
5.	Explained procedure to patient.	___	___	_____
6.	Washed hands and donned clean gloves.	___	___	_____
7.	Prepared patient for intervention.	___	___	_____
8.	Raised bed to comfortable working level.	___	___	_____
9.	Arranged for patient privacy.	___	___	_____
10.	Placed patient in Fowler's position.	___	___	_____
11.	Instructed patient to take three breaths and force cough into container.	___	___	_____
12.	Labeled specimen container.	___	___	_____
13.	Attached laboratory requisition and immediately took specimen to laboratory using a biohazard bag.	___	___	_____
14.	Removed gloves and washed hands.	___	___	_____
15.	Documented.	___	___	_____

**Performance Checklist
Skill 13–7**

OBTAINING A THROAT CULTURE

	S	U	Comments
1. Obtained equipment.	___	___	_____
2. Referred to medical record, care plan, or Kardex for special interventions.	___	___	_____
3. Introduced self.	___	___	_____
4. Identified patient by identification band.	___	___	_____
5. Explained procedure to patient.	___	___	_____
6. Washed hands and donned clean gloves.	___	___	_____
7. Prepared patient for intervention.	___	___	_____
8. Raised bed to comfortable working level.	___	___	_____
9. Arranged for patient privacy.	___	___	_____
10. Placed patient in sitting position unless contraindicated.	___	___	_____
11. Opened sterile swab.	___	___	_____
12. Requested patient to lean head back and to open mouth wide.	___	___	_____
13. Used tongue depressor if necessary.	___	___	_____
14. Gently but completely swabbed tonsillar region only from side to side and collected appropriate exudate or drainage.	___	___	_____
15. Placed swab in culturette.	___	___	_____
16. Replaced top on culturette.	___	___	_____
17. Discarded tongue depressor.	___	___	_____
18. Labeled specimen container.	___	___	_____
19. Attached laboratory requisition and immediately took specimen to laboratory in biohazard bag.	___	___	_____
20. Removed gloves and washed hands.	___	___	_____
21. Documented.	___	___	_____

**Performance Checklist
Skill 13–8**

ASSISTING WITH A PAPANICOLAOU TEST

	S	U	Comments
1. Obtained equipment.	___	___	_____
2. Referred to medical record, care plan, or Kardex for special interventions.	___	___	_____
3. Introduced self.	___	___	_____
4. Identified patient by identification band.	___	___	_____
5. Explained procedure to patient.	___	___	_____
6. Washed hands and donned clean gloves.	___	___	_____
7. Prepared patient for intervention.	___	___	_____
8. Raised bed to comfortable level.	___	___	_____
9. Arranged for patient privacy.	___	___	_____
10. Arranged for patient to empty bladder.	___	___	_____
11. Placed patient in lithotomy position.	___	___	_____
12. Draped patient.	___	___	_____
13. After physician completed the tests, cleansed equipment.	___	___	_____
14. Removed gloves and washed hands.	___	___	_____
15. Documented.	___	___	_____

**Performance Checklist
Skill 14–1**

PERFORMING A 2-MINUTE HANDWASHING

	S	U	Comments
1. Obtained equipment.			
2. Assessed hands, observing for visible dirt, breaks, and cuts in skin and cuticles.			
3. Determined contaminate of hands.			
4. Assessed areas around sink that are contaminated or clean.			
5. Removed jewelry and pushed watch and long sleeves above wrist.			
6. Adjusted water to right temperature and force.			
7. Wet hands and wrists thoroughly under warm running water, keeping hands lower than elbows.			
8. Lathered hands with liquid soap, about 1 teaspoon.			
9. Washed hands thoroughly using a firm circular motion and friction on back of hands, palms, and wrists, paying special attention to areas between fingers and knuckles by interlacing fingers and thumbs and moving hands back and forth.			
10. Washed 1 minute, rinsed thoroughly, relathered, and washed another minute using a continuous amount of friction.			
11. Rinsed wrists and hands completely, keeping hands lower than elbows.			
12. Cleansed fingernails thoroughly under running water using fingernails of other hand or blunt end of orange stick.			
13. Dried hands thoroughly with paper towels by patting dry at fingertips, hands, and then wrists and forearms.			
• Wet lower arms under running water. Washed lower arms with soap by completely circling arm for 10-15 seconds.			

	S	U	Comments

- Rinsed arms under running water, keeping hands and forearms lower than elbows. _____ _____ _____

- Washed hands again. _____ _____ _____

14. Turned off faucets with dry paper towel. _____ _____ _____

15. Used hand lotion if desired unless contraindicated. _____ _____ _____

16. Disposed of waste materials. _____ _____ _____

Performance Checklist
Skill 14–2

GLOVING

		S	U	Comments

1. Obtained equipment. ____ ____ _____

2. Washed and dried hands. ____ ____ _____

3. Assessed for need for gloves. ____ ____ _____

4. Removed gloves from dispenser. ____ ____ _____

5. Inspected gloves for possibility of perforation. ____ ____ _____

6. Donned gloves when ready to begin patient care. ____ ____ _____

7. If gloves were to be worn with gown, wore glove pulled up over cuffs of gown. ____ ____ _____

8. Changed gloves after direct handling of infectious drainage and did not touch side rails, tables, or stands with contaminated gloves. ____ ____ _____

9. Removed first glove by grasping at palm with other gloved hand and pulled glove off and inside out; placed this glove in opposite hand. ____ ____ _____

10. Removed second glove by placing finger under cuff edge and turned glove inside out and over other glove; dropped gloves into waste container. ____ ____ _____

11. Washed hands. ____ ____ _____

**Performance Checklist
Skill 14–3**

GOWNING FOR ISOLATION

	S	U	Comments
1. Obtained equipment.	___	___	_____
2. Determined need for use of isolation gown.	___	___	_____
3. Explained need for procedure to patient.	___	___	_____
4. Made certain patient informed that isolation procedure helps protect patient and nursing staff.	___	___	_____
5. Removed watch and pushed up long sleeves.	___	___	_____
6. Placed watch on paper towel or in plastic bag with closure before taking vital signs.	___	___	_____
7. Washed hands.	___	___	_____

Donning an isolation gown

	S	U	Comments
8. Opened gown by placing hands on inside of gown sleeves.	___	___	_____
9. Pulled gown on and securely tied gown at neck and then waist.	___	___	_____
10. Donned gloves and mask as necessary.	___	___	_____

Removing an isolation gown

	S	U	Comments
11. Untied waist ties first.	___	___	_____
12. Removed gloves.	___	___	_____
13. Untied neck ties next.	___	___	_____
14. Removed hands carefully from gown sleeves.	___	___	_____
15. Did not allow sleeves to be turned inside out to avoid touching outside of gown.	___	___	_____
16. Folded gown with outside surfaces touching.	___	___	_____
17. Disposed of gown in appropriate receptacle in room.	___	___	_____
18. Washed hands.	___	___	_____
19. Removed mask by untying.	___	___	_____
20. Disposed of waste in room.	___	___	_____

Performance Checklist
Skill 14–4

DONNING A MASK

	S	U	Comments
1. Obtained equipment.	___	___	_____
2. Washed hands.	___	___	_____
3. Removed mask from container.	___	___	_____
4. Chose appropriate mask for task.	___	___	_____

Donning mask

	S	U	Comments
5. Donned mask when ready to begin patient care by covering nose and mouth with mask.	___	___	_____
6. Secured mask in place with elastic band or tied strings at back of head.	___	___	_____
7. Wore mask until it became moist but no longer than 20 to 30 minutes.	___	___	_____

Removing mask

	S	U	Comments
8. Removed mask by untying strings or moving elastic, making certain not to touch contaminated area.	___	___	_____
9. Disposed of contaminated mask.	___	___	_____
10. Washed hands.	___	___	_____

**Performance Checklist
Skill 14–5**

PERFORMING DOUBLE BAGGING

	S	U	Comments
1. Obtained equipment.	___	___	_____
2. Washed hands.	___	___	_____
3. Donned gown, mask, and gloves before entering patient's room or performed double bagging before removing isolation garb following nursing care.	___	___	_____
4. Collected all contaminated disposable articles in isolation bag and tied securely without excess air.	___	___	_____
5. Summoned second health care worker to remain outside patient area.	___	___	_____
6. Second person held double bag with top edge of bag folded over to make clean edge covering hands.	___	___	_____
7. First person dropped contaminated bag in double bag without touching edges of bag.	___	___	_____
8. Sealed or tied and labeled bag.	___	___	_____
9. First person placed new bags in holder.	___	___	_____
10. Removed gown, gloves, and mask without contamination.	___	___	_____
11. Disposed of waste materials.	___	___	_____
12. Washed hands.	___	___	_____

Performance Checklist
Skill 14–6

PERFORMING ISOLATION TECHNIQUE

	S	U	Comments
1. Obtained equipment.	___	___	_____
2. Determined causative microorganism.	___	___	_____
3. Referred to medical record, care plan, or Kardex for special interventions.	___	___	_____
4. Introduced self.	___	___	_____
5. Identified patient by identification band.	___	___	_____
6. Explained procedure to patient.	___	___	_____
7. Prepared patient for intervention.	___	___	_____
8. Raised bed to comfortable working level.	___	___	_____
9. Arranged for patient privacy.	___	___	_____
10. Followed agency policy for type of isolation used.	___	___	_____
11. Posted isolation category instructions on door to room.	___	___	_____
12. Planned time to explain to patient and family.	___	___	_____
13. Washed hands and donned isolation garb according to agency policy.	___	___	_____
14. Provided required nursing care.	___	___	_____
15. Removed isolation garb and placed in isolation container.	___	___	_____
16. Disposed of waste materials.	___	___	_____
17. Removed gloves and washed hands.	___	___	_____
18. Documented.	___	___	_____

**Performance Checklist
Skill 14–7**

PREPARING FOR ANTISEPSIS, DISINFECTION, AND STERILIZATION

	S	U	Comments
1. Obtained equipment.	___	___	_____
2. Assessed contamination of article and need for cleansing, disinfection, or sterilization.	___	___	_____
3. Washed hands and donned clean gloves.	___	___	_____
4. Rinsed article under cold running water.	___	___	_____
5. Washed article under cold running water with appropriate agent.	___	___	_____
6. Used scrub brush to remove material in grooves.	___	___	_____
7. Dried article thoroughly.	___	___	_____
8. Prepared article for autoclave by wrapping in appropriate cloth wrappers.	___	___	_____
9. Disposed of waste materials.	___	___	_____
10. Removed gloves and washed hands.	___	___	_____

Performance Checklist
Skill 15–1

ADMINISTERING ORAL MEDICATIONS

	S	U	Comments
1. Obtained equipment.	___	___	_____
2. Compared medical order and medication profile.	___	___	_____
3. Washed hands before preparing medications.	___	___	_____
4. Compared label on medication container with medication profile.	___	___	_____
5. Read label second time before pouring tablets or liquids into dispensing cup.	___	___	_____
6. Prepared medication for one patient at a time.	___	___	_____
7. Opened unit dose medications at patient's bedside.	___	___	_____
8. Poured tablets and capsules from multidose drug containers into dispensing cup without touching medication.	___	___	_____
9. Poured liquid medication into appropriate-measured liquid medication cup and read dose at eye level.	___	___	_____
10. Palmed liquid medication away from label before pouring.	___	___	_____
11. Assessed by reading container a third time when returning medications to storage.	___	___	_____
12. Referred to medical record, care plan, of Kardex for special interventions.	___	___	_____
13. Introduced self.	___	___	_____
14. Identified patient by identification band.	___	___	_____
15. Explained procedure to patient.	___	___	_____
16. Washed hands and donned clean gloves.	___	___	_____
17. Assisted patient to sit up in bed unless contraindicated.	___	___	_____
18. Raised bed to comfortable working level.	___	___	_____

	S	U	Comments

19. Administered oral medications appropriately, making sure patient swallows every tablet or liquid.

20. Assisted patient to take medications, encouraging drinking plenty of water.

21. Remained at bedside until all medications were taken.

22. Removed gloves and washed hands.

23. Documented.

Performance Checklist
Skill 15–2

APPLYING A TRANSDERMAL MEDICATION PATCH

	S	U	Comments
1. Compared medication order with medication profile.	___	___	_____
2. Washed hands before preparing medications.	___	___	_____
3. Obtained equipment.	___	___	_____
4. Referred to medical record, care plan, or Kardex for special interventions.	___	___	_____
5. Introduced self.	___	___	_____
6. Identified patient by identification band.	___	___	_____
7. Explained procedure to patient.	___	___	_____
8. Washed hands and donned clean gloves.	___	___	_____
9. Prepared patient for intervention.	___	___	_____
10. Raised bed to comfortable working level.	___	___	_____
11. Arranged for patient privacy.	___	___	_____
12. Removed old patch and discarded in appropriate container.	___	___	_____
13. Cleansed old site with soap and water and dried well, observing for irritation, redness, and broken skin.	___	___	_____
14. Selected new site and cleansed and dried well.	___	___	_____
15. Peeled off patch backing, avoiding contact with drug.	___	___	_____
16. Pressed adhesive area of patch to skin until well adhered.	___	___	_____
17. Disposed of soiled supplies according to agency policy.	___	___	_____
18. Removed gloves and washed hands.	___	___	_____
19. Documented.	___	___	_____

Performance Checklist
Skill 15–3

ADMINISTERING EYE MEDICATIONS

		S	U	Comments
1.	Referred to medical record, care plan, or Kardex for special interventions.	___	___	_____
2.	Obtained equipment.	___	___	_____
3.	Compared medication order with medication profile.	___	___	_____
4.	Determined whether each eye would be treated differently.	___	___	_____
5.	Introduced self.	___	___	_____
6.	Identified patient by identification band.	___	___	_____
7.	Explained procedure to patient.	___	___	_____
8.	Washed hands and donned clean gloves.	___	___	_____
9.	Prepared patient for intervention.	___	___	_____
10.	Raised bed to comfortable working level.	___	___	_____
11.	Arranged for patient privacy.	___	___	_____
12.	Assessed condition of eyes.	___	___	_____
13.	Assisted to position of comfort with head tilted back.	___	___	_____
14.	Cleansed eye as necessary.	___	___	_____
15.	Gently pressed and pulled downward on bony prominence of eye.	___	___	_____
16.	Asked patient to look up and back toward ceiling.	___	___	_____
17.	Instill prescribed number of eyedrops into conjunctival sac of lower eyelid or applied thin stream of ointment across lower eyelid from inner to outer canthus.	___	___	_____
18.	Had patient close eye or eyes and gently moved eye from side to side and up and down.	___	___	_____
19.	Encouraged patient not to squint or squeeze eyes.	___	___	_____

	S	**U**	**Comments**

20. With medications that produce systemic effect, gently applied pressure to nasolacrimal duct for 30 to 60 seconds.

    ____ ____ _____

21. Gently wiped away excess medication from inner to outer canthus.

    ____ ____ _____

22. Applied pad or patch to eye if necessary.

    ____ ____ _____

23. Assisted patient to position of comfort and placed call bell within reach.

    ____ ____ _____

24. Removed gloves and washed hands.

    ____ ____ _____

25. Documented.

    ____ ____ _____

**Performance Checklist
Skill 15–4**

ADMINISTERING EAR MEDICATIONS

	S	U	Comments
1. Referred to medical record, care plan, or Kardex for special interventions.	____	____	_____
2. Obtained equipment.	____	____	_____
3. Compared medication order with medication profile.	____	____	_____
4. Warmed medication to body temperature.	____	____	_____
5. Introduced self.	____	____	_____
6. Identified patient by identification band.	____	____	_____
7. Explained procedure to patient.	____	____	_____
8. Washed hands and donned clean gloves.	____	____	_____
9. Prepared patient for intervention.	____	____	_____
10. Raised bed to comfortable working level.	____	____	_____
11. Arranged for patient privacy.	____	____	_____
12. Cleansed outer ear if needed.	____	____	_____
13. Assisted patient to position of comfort with affected ear directed toward ceiling.	____	____	_____
14. Appropriately straightened ear canal upward and back for adult or downward and back for young child.	____	____	_____
15. Held dropper $1/2$ inch above ear canal.	____	____	_____
16. Gently instilled prescribed number of drops onto side of ear canal.	____	____	_____
17. Encouraged patient to remain in position for 3 to 5 minutes.	____	____	_____
18. Allowed few minutes for medication to absorb before treating opposite ear.	____	____	_____
19. Treated opposite ear.	____	____	_____
20. Allowed opposite ear to absorb medication.	____	____	_____
21. Removed gloves and washed hands.	____	____	_____
22. Documented.	____	____	_____

**Performance Checklist
Skill 15–5**

ADMINISTERING RECTAL MEDICATIONS

		S	U	Comments
1.	Referred to medical record, care plan, or Kardex for special interventions.	____	____	_____
2.	Obtained equipment.	____	____	_____
3.	Compared medication order with medication profile.	____	____	_____
4.	Introduced self.	____	____	_____
5.	Identified patient by identification band.	____	____	_____
6.	Explained procedure to patient.	____	____	_____
7.	Washed hands and donned clean gloves.	____	____	_____
8.	Prepared patient for intervention.	____	____	_____
9.	Raised bed to comfortable working level.	____	____	_____
10.	Arranged for patient privacy.	____	____	_____
11.	Positioned patient on left side; exposed only buttocks.	____	____	_____
12.	Examined external anus for hemorrhoids and variations.	____	____	_____
13.	Removed suppository from wrapper and lubricated tip.	____	____	_____
14.	Asked patient to relax and breathe deeply with mouth open.	____	____	_____
15.	Assessed anus and gently inserted suppository past internal sphincter with index finger approximately 4 inches in an adult and 1 to 2 inches in an infant or a young child.	____	____	_____
16.	Withdrew finger and wiped anal area with tissue.	____	____	_____
17.	Assisted patient to retain suppository by holding buttocks together.	____	____	_____

	S	U	Comments

18. If suppository contained medication to facilitate defecation, placed call bell within reach or lowered side rails and placed bed in low position. _____ _____ _____

19. Removed gloves and washed hands. _____ _____ _____

20. Documented. _____ _____ _____

**Performance Checklist
Skill 15–6**

ADMINISTERING INJECTIONS

	S	U	Comments
1. Obtained equipment.	___	___	_____
2. Referred to medical record, care plan, or Kardex for special interventions.	___	___	_____
3. Introduced self.	___	___	_____
4. Identified patient by identification band.	___	___	_____
5. Explained procedure to patient.	___	___	_____
6. Washed hands and donned clean gloves.	___	___	_____
7. Prepared patient for intervention.	___	___	_____
8. Raised bed to comfortable working level.	___	___	_____
9. Arranged for patient privacy.	___	___	_____

Intradermal Injection

	S	U	Comments
10. Chose appropriate site and cleansed with alcohol swab.	___	___	_____
11. Stretched skin gently over site with thumb and index finger of nondominant hand.	___	___	_____
12. Inserted needle at 10- to 15-degree angle to forearm.	___	___	_____
13. Slid needle tip under skin where approximately 3-mm tip was visible through skin.	___	___	_____
14. Did not aspirate.	___	___	_____
15. Slowly injected medication, noting formation of bleb.	___	___	_____
16. Quickly removed needle.	___	___	_____
17. Did not massage site.	___	___	_____
18. Marked site with skin marker.	___	___	_____

Intramuscular Injection

	S	U	Comments
19. Using nondominant hand, spread skin tightly.	___	___	_____
20. With dominant hand, quickly darted needle into muscle at 90-degree angle.	___	___	_____

	S	U	Comments

21. Moved nondominant hand to stabilize syringe barrel near needle hub.

22. Aspirated.

23. Injected medication slowly until all medication was injected.

24. Applied pressure over site with antiseptic swab while withdrew needle quickly.

25. Massaged site with swab.

Subcutaneous Injection

26. With nondominant hand, gathered skin up between thumb and forefinger.

27. With dominant hand, quickly darted needle into tissue at 45- to 90-degree angle.

28. Moved nondominant hand to stabilize syringe by holding syringe barrel near needle hub.

29. Aspirated unless contraindicated.

30. Injected all medication slowly into subcutaneous tissue.

31. Removed needle quickly and applied pressure with antiseptic swab.

32. Massaged site to disperse medication.

33. Removed gloves and washed hands.

34. Documented.

**Performance Checklist
Skill 16–1**

INITIATING VENIPUNCTURE

	S	U	Comments
1. Obtained equipment.	___	___	_____
2. Referred to medical record, care plan, or Kardex for special interventions.	___	___	_____
3. Introduced self.	___	___	_____
4. Identified patient by identification band.	___	___	_____
5. Explained procedure to patient.	___	___	_____
6. Washed hands and donned clean gloves.	___	___	_____
7. Prepared patient for intervention.	___	___	_____
8. Raised bed to comfortable working level.	___	___	_____
9. Arranged for patient privacy.	___	___	_____
10. Identified venipuncture site.	___	___	_____
11. Applied tourniquet and selected venipuncture site.	___	___	_____
12. Cleansed site with appropriate agent using friction.	___	___	_____
13. Stretched skin and stabilized vein with nondominant hand.	___	___	_____
14. Holding angiocatheter bevel up, pierced skin above and slightly to side of vein at about a 45-degree angle.	___	___	_____
15. Lowered angle to 10 degrees and entered vein wall.	___	___	_____
16. Followed vein lumen with tip of needle to ensure placement within vein, assessing for blood return through angiocatheter backflow chamber.			
17. Released tourniquet.	___	___	_____
18. Holding guide needle in place, gently threaded plastic catheter off needle and into vein.	___	___	_____

	S	U	Comments

19. Applying gentle pressure over catheter in vein, removed guide needle and attached sterile connection end of primed tubing into catheter hub.

20. Stabilizing insertion site, slowly opened flow valve to begin intravenous infusion.

21. Following agency policy, secured and dressed site with tape, medication, and dressing.

22. Labeled site and tubing according to agency policy.

23. Adjusted fluid flow rate according to accurate drop rate calculations.

24. Removed gloves and washed hands.

25. Documented.

**Performance Checklist
Skill 16–2**

ADMINISTERING BLOOD

		S	U	Comments
1.	Assessed for informed consent form.			
2.	Obtained equipment.			
3.	Referred to medical record, care plan, or Kardex for special interventions.			
4.	Introduced self.			
5.	Identified patient by identification band.			
6.	Explained procedure to patient.			
7.	Washed hands and donned clean gloves.			
8.	Prepared patient for intervention.			
9.	Raised bed to comfortable working level.			
10.	Arranged for patient privacy.			
11.	Initiated primary intravenous infusion or hung 0.9% normal saline container and flushed tubing into existing intravenous infusion.			
12.	Obtained blood just before infusing.			
13.	Verified blood compatibility and patient identity according to agency policy.			
14.	Attached filtered blood-administration tubing to blood unit container and primed.			
15.	Piggybacked blood-filled tubing to Y site closest to patient.			
16.	Obtained baseline vital signs.			
17.	Began transfusion slowly.			
18.	Took vital signs every 5 minutes for 15 minutes.			
19.	If reaction symptoms occurred, stopped transfusion and followed steps of nursing interventions for transfusion reaction.			
20.	Instructed patient to immediately report any rash, itching, chills, or headache.			

	S	U	Comments
21. Adjusted flow rate using infusion pump.	___	___	_____
22. Observed and assessed patient frequently according to agency policy.	___	___	_____
23. Discontinued blood transfusion when blood infused: maintained primary intravenous infusion of 0.9% normal saline.	___	___	_____
24. Removed gloves and washed hands.	___	___	_____
25. Documented.	___	___	_____

Performance Checklist
Skill 16–3

ADMINISTERING CHEMOTHERAPY

	S	U	Comments
1. Obtained equipment.	___	___	_____
2. Referred to medical record, care plan, or Kardex for special interventions.	___	___	_____
3. Introduced self.	___	___	_____
4. Identified patient by identification band.	___	___	_____
5. Explained procedure to patient.	___	___	_____
6. Washed hands and donned clean gloves.	___	___	_____
7. Prepared patient for intervention.	___	___	_____
8. Raised bed to comfortable working level.	___	___	_____
9. Arranged for patient privacy.	___	___	_____
10. Verified informed consent.	___	___	_____
11. Reviewed laboratory reports and recorded current patient history and vital signs; provided patient opportunity to discuss feelings.	___	___	_____
12. Read medical order and medication label 3 times and verified dosage, medication, and patient.	___	___	_____
13. Administered preventative measures as ordered.	___	___	_____
14. Donned sterile gloves.	___	___	_____
15. Placed emergency equipment and medications nearby.	___	___	_____
16. Performed venipuncture or verified placement of intravenous infusion or heparin/saline lock by assessing for blood return.	___	___	_____
17. Cleansed injection port and inserted stopcock device.	___	___	_____
18. Inserted syringe or piggyback tubing connection into stopcock device.	___	___	_____
19. Slowly began to infuse medication.	___	___	_____

106

20. Administered medication by pump or volume-control device, aspirating and assessing patient response frequently. ____ ____ _____

21. Stopped chemotherapy immediately if severe reaction or extravasation occurred. ____ ____ _____

22. Flushed intravenous infusion lines between multiple medication administration. ____ ____ _____

23. Frequently observed and assessed infusion and patient. ____ ____ _____

24. When medication was completely infused, removed piggyback tubing and container or syringe and disposed of according to agency policy in biohazard containers. ____ ____ _____

25. Removed protective gear and disposed of according to agency policy. ____ ____ _____

26. Instructed patient on disposal of body fluids for next 48 hours. ____ ____ _____

27. Removed gloves and washed hands. ____ ____ _____

28. Documented. ____ ____ _____

**Performance Checklist
Skill 17–1**

TEACHING POSTOPERATIVE BREATHING TECHNIQUES AND LEG EXERCISES

	S	U	Comments
1. Obtained equipment.	___	___	_____
2. Referred to medical record, care plan, or Kardex for special interventions.	___	___	_____
3. Introduced self.	___	___	_____
4. Identified patient by identification band.	___	___	_____
5. Explained procedure to patient.	___	___	_____
6. Washed hands and donned clean gloves.	___	___	_____
7. Prepared patient for intervention.	___	___	_____
8. Raised bed to comfortable working level.	___	___	_____
9. Arranged for patient privacy.	___	___	_____
10. Premedicated with pain medication if indicated.	___	___	_____

Deep Breathing Exercises

	S	U	Comments
11. Placed pillow between patient and bed or chair.	___	___	_____
12. Sat or stood facing patient.	___	___	_____
13. Demonstrated taking slow, deep breaths, avoiding using shoulder and chest while inhaling; inhaled through nose.	___	___	_____
14. Held breath for count of 3 and slowly exhaled through pursed lips.	___	___	_____
15. Repeated exercise 3 to 5 times; had patient practice exercise.	___	___	_____
16. Instructed patient to take 10 slow breaths every 2 hours after surgery during waking hours until ambulatory.	___	___	_____
17. If patient has an abdominal or a chest incision, instructed to splint incisional area if desired during breathing exercises.	___	___	_____

	S	**U**	**Comments**

Leg Exercises

18. Lifting one leg at a time and supporting joints, gently flexed and extended leg 5 to 10 times.

19. Repeated exercise with opposite leg. Lifting leg while supporting joints, gently flexed and extended leg 5 to 10 times.

20. Alternately pointed toes toward chin and toward foot of bed 4 to 5 times.

21. Made circles with ankles of both feet 4 to 5 times to left and 4 to 5 times to right.

22. Assessed pulse, respiration, and blood pressure.

23. Removed gloves and washed hands.

24. Documented.

**Performance Checklist
Skill 17–2**

TEACHING CONTROLLED COUGHING

		S	U	Comments
1.	Obtained equipment.	___	___	_____
2.	Referred to medical record, care plan, or Kardex for special interventions.	___	___	_____
3.	Introduced self.	___	___	_____
4.	Identified patient by identification band.	___	___	_____
5.	Explained procedure to patient.	___	___	_____
6.	Washed hands and donned clean gloves.	___	___	_____
7.	Prepared patient for intervention.	___	___	_____
8.	Raised bed to comfortable working level.	___	___	_____
9.	Arranged for patient privacy.	___	___	_____
10.	Premedicated with pain medication if indicated.	___	___	_____
11.	Assisted patient to an upright position; placed pillow between bed and chair and patient.	___	___	_____
12.	Explained importance of maintaining an upright position.	___	___	_____
13.	Demonstrated coughing exercise for patient.	___	___	_____
14.	Splinted abdominal or thoracic incision with hands, pillow, folded towel, or folded bath blanket before coughing if desired.	___	___	_____
15.	Encouraged patient to practice coughing while splinting incisional area once or twice an hour during waking hours.	___	___	_____
16.	Provided tissue and emesis basin for phlegm, secretions, and mucus expectorated.	___	___	_____
17.	Provided washcloth and warm water for washing hands and face and returned patient to comfortable position.	___	___	_____
18.	Cleansed emesis basin and appropriately disposed of tissues.	___	___	_____
19.	Removed gloves and washed hands.	___	___	_____
20.	Documented.	___	___	_____

**Performance Checklist
Skill 17–3**

PERFORMING A SURGICAL SHAVE

		S	U	Comments
1.	Obtained equipment.	___	___	_____
2.	Referred to medical record, care plan, or Kardex for special interventions.	___	___	_____
3.	Introduced self.	___	___	_____
4.	Identified patient by identification band.	___	___	_____
5.	Explained procedure to patient.	___	___	_____
6.	Washed hands and donned clean gloves.	___	___	_____
7.	Prepared patient for intervention.	___	___	_____
8.	Raised bed to comfortable working level.	___	___	_____
9.	Arranged for patient privacy.	___	___	_____
10.	Positioned bed and patient.	___	___	_____
11.	Placed towel or waterproof pad under area to be shaved.	___	___	_____
12.	Filled basin with warm water.	___	___	_____
13.	Placed bath blanket over patient.	___	___	_____
14.	Adjusted lighting.	___	___	_____
15.	Lathered skin with antiseptic soap and warm water using gauze squares.	___	___	_____
16.	Held razor at 30- to 45-degree angle to skin and shaved patient.	___	___	_____
17.	Rinsed razor frequently.	___	___	_____
18.	When entire area was shaved, used washcloth and clean, warm water to cleanse area; dried skin.	___	___	_____
19.	Reassessed skin for cuts, nicks, and hair.	___	___	_____
20.	Returned patient to appropriate position.	___	___	_____
21.	Cleansed and disposed of equipment.	___	___	_____
22.	Removed gloves and washed hands.	___	___	_____
23.	Documented.	___	___	_____

Performance Checklist
Skill 17–4

MAKING A SURGICAL BED

	S	U	Comments
1. Obtained equipment.	___	___	_____
2. Referred to medical record, care plan, or Kardex for special interventions.	___	___	_____
3. Introduced self.	___	___	_____
4. Identified patient by identification band.	___	___	_____
5. Explained procedure to patient.	___	___	_____
6. Washed hands and donned clean gloves.	___	___	_____
7. Prepared patient for intervention.	___	___	_____
8. Raised bed to comfortable working level.	___	___	_____
9. Arranged for patient privacy.	___	___	_____
10. Examined room to determine to which side of bed patient will be returned.	___	___	_____
11. Placed linens within easy reach.	___	___	_____
12. Stripped bed according to procedure in Chapter 23.	___	___	_____
13. Made foundation of bed according to procedure in Chapter 23.	___	___	_____
14. Placed bath blanket or flannel sheet on foundation bed if called for in agency policy.	___	___	_____
15. Placed disposable pad or towel for patient's head (optional).	___	___	_____
16. Placed top sheet and spread on bed, leaving both untucked.	___	___	_____
17. Folded top linens down about 6 inches from top of bed and up 6 inches from bottom of bed.	___	___	_____
18. Fanfolded top sheets according to agency policy.	___	___	_____
19. Changed pillow case and placed pillow on bedside chair.	___	___	_____

	S	U	Comments
20. Locked wheels of bed.	____	____	_____
21. Left bed in high position.	____	____	_____
22. Placed emesis basin and tissues at bedside.	____	____	_____
23. Provided any other equipment ordered by physician.	____	____	_____
24. Discarded dirty linen and tidied room.	____	____	_____
25. Removed gloves and washed hands.	____	____	_____
26. Documented.	____	____	_____

Performance Checklist
Skill 17–5

RECEIVING THE PATIENT FROM THE POSTANESTHESIA CARE UNIT

	S	U	Comments
1. Obtained equipment.	___	___	_____
2. Referred to medical record, care plan, or Kardex for special interventions.	___	___	_____
3. Introduced self.	___	___	_____
4. Identified patient by identification band.	___	___	_____
5. Explained procedure to patient.	___	___	_____
6. Washed hands and donned clean gloves.	___	___	_____
7. Prepared patient for intervention.	___	___	_____
8. Raised bed to comfortable working level.	___	___	_____
9. Arranged for patient privacy.	___	___	_____
10. Determined time of arrival on unit.	___	___	_____
11. Transferred patient to surgical bed.	___	___	_____
12. Placed patient on side unless contraindicated or turned head to one side.	___	___	_____
13. Assessed level of consciousness.	___	___	_____
14. Assessed patent airway.	___	___	_____
15. Obtained vital signs.	___	___	_____
16. Assessed skin color and condition for diaphoresis; cool, clammy skin; pallor; and cyanosis.	___	___	_____
17. Assessed dressings for bleeding and drainage.	___	___	_____
18. Assessed intravenous infusion and assessed site.	___	___	_____
19. Read medical orders for further instructions.	___	___	_____
20. Assessed tubes and drains for patency.	___	___	_____
21. Assessed patient for pain and discomfort.	___	___	_____

	S	U	Comments
22. Raised side rails, lowered bed, and placed call light within reach of patient.	____	____	_____
23. Communicated with family.	____	____	_____
24. Removed gloves and washed hands.	____	____	_____
25. Documented.	____	____	_____

Performance Checklist
Skill 17–6

APPLYING ANTIEMBOLISM STOCKINGS

	S	U	Comments
1. Obtained equipment.	___	___	_____
2. Referred to medical record, care plan, or Kardex for special interventions.	___	___	_____
3. Introduced self.	___	___	_____
4. Identified patient by identification band.	___	___	_____
5. Explained procedure to patient.	___	___	_____
6. Washed hands and donned clean gloves.	___	___	_____
7. Prepared patient for intervention.	___	___	_____
8. Raised bed to comfortable working level.	___	___	_____
9. Arranged for patient privacy.	___	___	_____
10. Examined legs and assessed for high-risk conditions.	___	___	_____
11. Assessed patient for calf pain and positive Homan's sign.	___	___	_____
12. Measured legs for stockings according to agency policy and ordered stockings.	___	___	_____

Antiembolism stockings

	S	U	Comments
13. Assisted patient to supine position.	___	___	_____
14. Turned stocking inside out as far as heel; placed thumbs inside foot part, and slipped stocking on until heel is correctly aligned.	___	___	_____
15. Gathered up fabric and eased it over ankle and up leg.	___	___	_____
16. Pulled leg portion of stocking over foot and up as far as it would go (groin), making certain gusset lies over femoral artery; adjusted stocking to fit evenly and smoothly with no wrinkles.	___	___	_____
17. Repeat procedure for opposite leg.	___	___	_____

	S	U	Comments

Sequential Compression Device (SCD)

18. Placed sleeve under patient's leg with fuller portion at top of thigh.

19. Applied sleeve with opening at front of knee and closed portion behind knee.

20. When in place, made sure there were no wrinkles or creases in stockings and folded Velcro strips over to secure stockings in place.

21. Attached tubing to SCD after both sleeves were applied, with arrows needing to be aligned for correct connection and appropriate effect; plugged in unit.

22. Assessed patient periodically.

23. Assessed stockings at regular intervals.

24. Removed gloves and washed hands.

25. Documented.

Performance Checklist
Skill 17–7

APPLYING HEAT

	S	U	Comments

1. Obtained equipment.

2. Referred to medical record, care plan, or Kardex for special interventions.

3. Introduced self.

4. Identified patient by identification band.

5. Explained procedure to patient.

6. Washed hands and donned clean gloves.

7. Prepared patient for intervention.

8. Raised bed to comfortable working level.

9. Arranged for patient privacy.

10. Exposed only area to be treated.

Hot Water Bottle

11. Measured temperature of water.

12. Filled bottle one-third to one-half full.

13. Expelled air from bottle.

14. Secured stopper.

15. Assessed for leaks.

16. Dried bottle and applied cover.

17. Applied to treatment area.

18. Assessed treatment area every 10 minutes or according to agency policy.

19. Allowed heat to remain on affected area for approximately 30 minutes or as ordered by physician.

Heat Lamp

20. Assessed patient's skin to make sure it is clean and dry.

21. Positioned lamp at appropriate angle and 18 to 24 inches from area to be treated (by measurement) with bulb no greater than 60 watts.

	S	U	Comments

22. Did not cover lamp. ___ ___ _____

23. Assessed patient at least every 10 minutes. ___ ___ _____

24. Removed lamp at appropriate time or according to agency policy. ___ ___ _____

Warm Compresses

25. Positioned patient in comfortable position. ___ ___ _____

26. Prepared appropriate solution. ___ ___ _____

27. Saturated gauze or clean washcloth in solution and wrung excess solution from gauze or washcloth. ___ ___ _____

28. Placed gauze or washcloth slowly over area to be treated. ___ ___ _____

29. Covered gauze or washcloth with dry towel and piece of plastic. ___ ___ _____

30. Secured compress with tape or ties. ___ ___ _____

31. Applied warming device to outer cover if required; assessed skin frequently, at least every 10 minutes. ___ ___ _____

32. Remoistened gauze as needed to keep it warm. ___ ___ _____

33. After appropriate time, removed gauze or washcloth and disposed of appropriately. ___ ___ _____

34. Removed gloves and washed hands. ___ ___ _____

35. Documented. ___ ___ _____

Performance Checklist
Skill 17–8

APPLYING COLD

		S	U	Comments
1.	Obtained equipment.	___	___	_____
2.	Referred to medical record, care plan, or Kardex for special interventions.	___	___	_____
3.	Introduced self.	___	___	_____
4.	Identified patient by identification band.	___	___	_____
5.	Explained procedure to patient.	___	___	_____
6.	Washed hands and donned clean gloves.	___	___	_____
7.	Prepared patient for intervention.	___	___	_____
8.	Raised bed to comfortable working level.	___	___	_____
9.	Arranged for patient privacy.	___	___	_____
10.	Positioned patient in comfortable position with only treatment area exposed.	___	___	_____

Ice Bag

		S	U	Comments
11.	Filled bag one-third to one-half full of crushed ice.	___	___	_____
12.	Expelled excess air.	___	___	_____
13.	Secured stopper.	___	___	_____
14.	Assessed for leaks.	___	___	_____
15.	Dried bottle and applied cover.	___	___	_____
16.	Applied to treatment area.	___	___	_____
17.	Assessed treatment area every 5 to 10 minutes.	___	___	_____
18.	Allowed to remain in place for appropriate time or as ordered by physician.	___	___	_____

Ice Collar

		S	U	Comments
19.	If ice collar needs to be refilled, followed first five steps as with ice bag.	___	___	_____
20.	If prefilled ice bag is used, removed from freezer and applied cover.	___	___	_____

	S	U	Comments

21. Positioned ice collar on patient. ____ ____ _____

22. Secured with roller gauze or binder, tape, or safety pins; avoided puncturing collar with safety pin. ____ ____ _____

23. Assessed patient every 5 to 10 minutes; assessed temperature of ice collar. ____ ____ _____

24. Removed ice collar at appropriate time. ____ ____ _____

Cold Compresses

25. Prepared appropriate solution. ____ ____ _____

26. Saturated gauze or clean washcloth in solution. ____ ____ _____

27. Wrung excess solution from gauze or washcloth. ____ ____ _____

28. Placed gauze or washcloth over area to be treated. ____ ____ _____

29. Covered gauze or washcloth with dry towel or waterproof pad. ____ ____ _____

30. Secured in place with ties or tape. ____ ____ _____

31. Applied to outside surface of compress. ____ ____ _____

32. Assessed skin frequently at least every 10 minutes. ____ ____ _____

33. Remoistened compress as needed. ____ ____ _____

34. Removed compress at appropriate time and disposed of according to agency policy. ____ ____ _____

Ice Mattress (Hypothermic Blanket)

35. Prepared pad or blanket. ____ ____ _____

36. Took patient's temperature. ____ ____ _____

37. Placed one bath blanket beneath patient and over cooling pad and one bath blanket over patient. ____ ____ _____

38. Connected pad/blanket to cooling unit. ____ ____ _____

39. Plugged in unit. ____ ____ _____

40. Took temperature frequently. ____ ____ _____

41. Removed blanket when desired body temperature was reached or according to agency policy. ____ ____ _____

Chemical Pack

42. Activated chemical reaction by squeezing or kneading action. ____ ____ _____

43. Covered with cloth if needed. ____ ____ _____

Performance Checklist
Skill 17–8

APPLYING COLD (Continued)

	S	U	Comments
44. Assessed skin and temperature of pack every 5 to 10 minutes.	___	___	_____
45. Removed after treatment was completed.	___	___	_____
46. Placed patient in comfortable position after treatment.	___	___	_____
47. Disposed of or cleaned and returned equipment to appropriate storage or for cleaning.	___	___	_____
48. Removed gloves and washed hands.	___	___	_____
49. Documented.	___	___	_____

Performance Checklist
Skill 17–9

CARING FOR SURGICAL DRAINS

	S	U	Comments
1. Obtained equipment.	___	___	_____
2. Referred to medical record, care plan, or Kardex for special interventions.	___	___	_____
3. Introduced self.	___	___	_____
4. Identified patient by identification band.	___	___	_____
5. Explained procedure to patient.	___	___	_____
6. Washed hands and donned clean gloves.	___	___	_____
7. Prepared patient for intervention.	___	___	_____
8. Raised bed to comfortable working level.	___	___	_____
9. Arranged for patient privacy.	___	___	_____
10. Premedicated with pain medication if indicated.	___	___	_____
11. Asked patient not to touch drain site.	___	___	_____
12. Placed soiled dressing in moisture-proof bag; removed gloves and discarded.	___	___	_____
13. Wash hands and donned clean gloves.	___	___	_____
14. Poured antiseptic solution into sterile container.	___	___	_____
15. Placed sterile gauze squares in solution and removed contaminated gloves.	___	___	_____
16. Donned sterile gloves.	___	___	_____
17. Squeezed excess solution out of gauze square and cleansed drain site.	___	___	_____
18. Placed sterile, precut, split 4 x 4 drain gauze around drain.	___	___	_____
19. Applied sterile dressing if appropriate; avoided kinking tubing.	___	___	_____

	S	U	Comments

20. Placed graduated container under outlet of closed drainage-collection container; removed cap or clamp, and poured contents into graduate; assessed drainage, noted measurement, and discarded.   ____ ____ _____

21. Removed gloves and washed hands.   ____ ____ _____

22. Documented.   ____ ____ _____

Performance Checklist
Skill 17–10

APPLYING A BANDAGE

	S	U	Comments
1. Obtained equipment.	___	___	_____
2. Referred to medical record, care plan, or Kardex for special interventions.	___	___	_____
3. Introduced self.	___	___	_____
4. Identified patient by identification band.	___	___	_____
5. Explained procedure to patient.	___	___	_____
6. Washed hands and donned clean gloves.	___	___	_____
7. Prepared patient for intervention.	___	___	_____
8. Raised bed to comfortable working level.	___	___	_____
9. Arranged for patient privacy.	___	___	_____
10. Premedicated with pain medication if indicated.	___	___	_____
11. Positioned patient in comfortable position, arranging support for area to be bandaged.	___	___	_____
12. Ensured that skin and dressing were clean and dry.	___	___	_____
13. Separated any adjacent skin surfaces.	___	___	_____
14. Aligned part to be bandaged, providing slight flexion if appropriate and not contraindicated.	___	___	_____
15. Applied bandage from distal to proximal part.	___	___	_____
16. Applied bandage with even distribution of pressure.	___	___	_____

Use appropriate bandage turns

	S	U	Comments
17. Use circular, spiral, spiral-reverse, recurrent (stump), or figure-eight.	___	___	_____
18. Positioned patient for comfort.	___	___	_____
19. Removed gloves and washed hands.	___	___	_____
20. Documented.	___	___	_____

**Performance Checklist
Skill 17–11**

APPLYING A BINDER, ARM SLING, OR T–BINDER

	S	**U**	**Comments**
1. Obtained equipment.	___	___	_____
2. Referred to medical record, care plan, or Kardex for special interventions.	___	___	_____
3. Introduced self.	___	___	_____
4. Identified patient by identification band.	___	___	_____
5. Explained procedure to patient.	___	___	_____
6. Washed hands and donned clean gloves.	___	___	_____
7. Prepared patient for intervention.	___	___	_____
8. Raised bed to comfortable working level.	___	___	_____
9. Arranged for patient privacy.	___	___	_____
10. Premedicated with pain medication if indicated.	___	___	_____
11. Assisted patient to comfortable position.	___	___	_____
12. Changed dressing if appropriate and washed skin if needed.	___	___	_____
13. Separated skin surfaces or padded bony prominences.	___	___	_____
14. Applied Velcro binder by placing it under patient's waist and hips, pulling it tight but not constricting.	___	___	_____

Triangular binder (sling)

	S	**U**	**Comments**
15. Had patient flex arm at approximately 80-degree angle depending on purpose.	___	___	_____
16. Placed end of triangular binder over shoulder of injured side (front to back).	___	___	_____
17. Picked up other end of binder and brought it up and over injured arm to shoulder of injured arm.	___	___	_____
18. Used a square knot to tie two ends together at side of neck on injured side.	___	___	_____

	S	**U**	**Comments**

19. Supported wrist well with binder; did not allow it to hang down over end of binder.

_____ _____ _____

20. Folded third triangle end neatly around elbow and secured with safety pins.

_____ _____ _____

T-Bandage

21. Using appropriate binder, placed waistband smoothly under waist of patient; tails should have been under patient.

_____ _____ _____

22. Secured two ends of waistband together with safety pin.

_____ _____ _____

23. For single tail, brought tail up between legs to secure dressing in place.

_____ _____ _____

24. For two tails, brought tails up, one on each side of penis or large dressing.

_____ _____ _____

25. Brought tails under and over waistband and secured with safety pins.

_____ _____ _____

26. Removed gloves and washed hands.

_____ _____ _____

27. Documented.

_____ _____ _____

Performance Checklist
Skill 18–1

PERFORMING STERILE GLOVE TECHNIQUE (OPEN GLOVING)

	S	U	Comments
1. Obtained equipment.	___	___	_____
2. Placed package of sterile gloves on a clean, dry surface at waist level or above.	___	___	_____
3. Carefully peeled back outer wrapper of glove package.	___	___	_____
4. Opened inner package (wrapper) with cuff ends of gloves facing self; did not touch inside of wrapper.	___	___	_____
5. With thumb and index finger of nondominant hand, picked up folded cuff of glove for dominant hand.	___	___	_____
6. Held glove with fingers facing slightly upward and lifted up and away from wrapper.	___	___	_____
7. Carefully inserted dominant hand into glove without touching outside of glove.	___	___	_____
8. Inserted fingers of gloved hand under cuff of second glove, keeping thumb away from hand; picked glove up away from sterile wrapper.	___	___	_____
9. Inserted nondominant hand into glove, being careful not to touch gloved hand with ungloved hand.	___	___	_____
10. Adjusted fit of both gloves, especially smoothing fingers, touching only outer surfaces of both gloves.	___	___	_____
11. To remove gloves, grasped glove of nondominant hand near cuff and removed by inverting glove; collected contaminated glove in gloved hand and wad into a fist.	___	___	_____

	S	U	Comments

12. Slid fingers of ungloved hand inside opposite glove and removed by turning inside out and pulling over both gloves. ___ ___ _____

13. Disposed gloves. ___ ___ _____

14. Washed hands. ___ ___ _____

Performance Checklist
Skill 18–2

PERFORMING STERILE DRESSING CHANGE

	S	U	Comments
1. Obtained equipment.	___	___	_____
2. Referred to medical record, care plan, or Kardex for special interventions.	___	___	_____
3. Introduced self.	___	___	_____
4. Identified patient by identification band.	___	___	_____
5. Explained procedure to patient.	___	___	_____
6. Washed hands and donned clean gloves.	___	___	_____
7. Prepared patient for intervention.	___	___	_____
8. Raised bed to working level.	___	___	_____
9. Arranged for patient privacy.	___	___	_____
10. Placed refuse container in convenient location away from sterile field.	___	___	_____
11. Set up sterile field.	___	___	_____
12. Loosened tapes by pulling toward incision and gently pulling skin away from tape.	___	___	_____
13. Removed soiled dressing and discarded.	___	___	_____
14. Assessed status of wound and wound drainage on dressing.	___	___	_____
15. Removed gloves, washed hands, and donned sterile gloves.	___	___	_____
16. Cleansed wound and surrounding area with antiseptic swabs, starting from incision outward, one stroke with each swab.	___	___	_____
17. Cleansed drain site if applicable.	___	___	_____
18. Applied special order ointment if applicable.	___	___	_____
19. Covered wound with appropriately sized dry sterile dressing and used drain dressing if applicable.	___	___	_____
20. Applied bandage, secured with tape, Montgomery straps, or binder.	___	___	_____

21. Removed sterile gloves and donned clean gloves.

___ ___ _____

22. Discarded refuse in biohazard bag.

___ ___ _____

23. Repositioned patient.

___ ___ _____

24. Removed gloves and washed hands.

___ ___ _____

25. Documented.

___ ___ _____

**Performance Checklist
Skill 18–3**

OBTAINING A STERILE WOUND CULTURE

		S	U	Comments
1.	Obtained equipment.	___	___	_____
2.	Referred to medical record, care plan, or Kardex for special interventions.	___	___	_____
3.	Introduced self.	___	___	_____
4.	Identified patient by identification band.	___	___	_____
5.	Explained procedure to patient.	___	___	_____
6.	Washed hands and donned clean gloves.	___	___	_____
7.	Prepared patient for intervention.	___	___	_____
8.	Raised bed to comfortable working level.	___	___	_____
9.	Arranged for patient privacy.	___	___	_____
10.	Positioned patient.	___	___	_____
11.	Placed refuse container in convenient location away from sterile field.	___	___	_____
12.	Set up sterile field.	___	___	_____
13.	Loosened dressing tape by pulling toward incision and using thumb, gently pulling skin away from tape.	___	___	_____
14.	Using clean gloves, removed dressing and discarded into refuse bag.	___	___	_____
15.	Assessed status of wound and wound drainage on dressing.	___	___	_____
16.	Removed gloves, washed hands, and donned sterile gloves.	___	___	_____
17.	Cleansed wound and surrounding area with antiseptic swabs and discarded.	___	___	_____
18.	Removed sterile culture swab from culture tube and gently inserted into drainage or into wound itself.	___	___	_____
19.	Removed swab from wound and inserted into sterile culture tube.	___	___	_____

	S	U	Comments

20. Crushed ampule of culture medium at bottom of tube and pushed swab into fluid. ____ ____ _____

21. Put cap or lid on culture tube tightly. ____ ____ _____

22. Cleansed wound with antiseptic swabs and applied sterile dressing. ____ ____ _____

23. Removed sterile gloves and donned clean gloves. ____ ____ _____

24. Discarded refuse appropriately. ____ ____ _____

25. Labeled culture specimen with exact location of culture source and sent promptly to laboratory with requisition. ____ ____ _____

26. Removed gloves and washed hands. ____ ____ _____

27. Documented. ____ ____ _____

**Performance Checklist
Skill 18–4**

APPLYING A WET-TO-DRY DRESSING

	S	U	Comments
1. Obtained equipment.	___	___	_____
2. Referred to medical record, care plan, or Kardex for special interventions.	___	___	_____
3. Introduced self.	___	___	_____
4. Identified patient by identification band.	___	___	_____
5. Explained procedure to patient.	___	___	_____
6. Washed hands and donned clean gloves.	___	___	_____
7. Prepared patient for intervention.	___	___	_____
8. Raised bed to comfortable working level.	___	___	_____
9. Arranged for patient privacy.	___	___	_____
10. Positioned patient.	___	___	_____
11. Placed waterproof pad appropriately.	___	___	_____
12. Placed refuse container appropriately.	___	___	_____
13. Set up sterile field.	___	___	_____
14. Loosened tape by pulling toward incision and using thumb, gently pulling skin away from tape.	___	___	_____
15. Removed dressing and discarded into refuse bag.	___	___	_____
16. Assessed status of wound and wound drainage on dressing.	___	___	_____
17. Removed gloves, washed hands, and donned sterile gloves.	___	___	_____
18. Cleansed wound from incision outward, one stroke with each swab, and discarded.	___	___	_____
19. Placed gauze into basin.	___	___	_____
20. Wrung excess solution from dressing, leaving it slightly moist.	___	___	_____
21. Placed gauze over open wound surfaces and pressed into depressed areas.	___	___	_____

	S	U	Comments

22. Applied dry dressing over wet gauze.   ____ ____ _____

23. Covered with additional dressing as needed. ____ ____ _____

24. Secured with tape or Montgomery straps. ____ ____ _____

25. Removed sterile gloves, washed hands, and donned clean gloves. ____ ____ _____

26. Repositioned patient. ____ ____ _____

27. Discarded refuse appropriately in biohazard bag. ____ ____ _____

28. Removed gloves and washed hands. ____ ____ _____

29. Documented. ____ ____ _____

**Performance Checklist
Skill 18–5**

APPLYING A STERILE COMPRESS

	S	U	Comments
1. Obtained equipment.	___	___	_____
2. Referred to medical record, care plan, or Kardex for special interventions.	___	___	_____
3. Introduced self.	___	___	_____
4. Identified patient by identification band.	___	___	_____
5. Explained procedure to patient.	___	___	_____
6. Washed hands and donned clean gloves.	___	___	_____
7. Prepared patient for intervention.	___	___	_____
8. Raised bed to comfortable working level.	___	___	_____
9. Arranged for patient privacy.	___	___	_____
10. Positioned patient.	___	___	_____
11. Placed refuse container in convenient location away from sterile field.	___	___	_____
12. Set up sterile field.	___	___	_____
13. Removed outer tape gently.	___	___	_____
14. Removed dressing and discarded in refuse container.	___	___	_____
15. Assessed wound status and wound drainage on dressing.	___	___	_____
16. Washed hands and donned clean gloves.	___	___	_____
17. Cleansed wound and surrounding area with antiseptic swab.	___	___	_____
18. Wrung out solution-soaked gauze and applied to total wound area.	___	___	_____
19. Covered compress with sterile drape.	___	___	_____
20. Applied aquathermic device over drape for 20 to 30 minutes.	___	___	_____
21. Monitored patient frequently during procedure and inspected site.	___	___	_____

	S	U	Comments

22. Removed gloves and discarded soiled dressings. ___ ___ _____

23. Repositioned patient. ___ ___ _____

24. Removed compress in 30 minutes or as ordered, using clean gloves; discarded appropriately. ___ ___ _____

25. Assessed wound and surrounding skin. ___ ___ _____

26. Donned sterile gloves. ___ ___ _____

27. Redressed wound if applicable. ___ ___ _____

28. Removed gloves and washed hands. ___ ___ _____

29. Documented. ___ ___ _____

**Performance Checklist
Skill 18–6**

PERFORMING STERILE IRRIGATION

	S	U	Comments
1. Obtained equipment.	___	___	_____
2. Referred to medical record, care plan, or Kardex for special interventions.	___	___	_____
3. Introduced self.	___	___	_____
4. Identified patient by identification band.	___	___	_____
5. Explained procedure to patient	___	___	_____
6. Washed hands and donned clean gloves.	___	___	_____
7. Prepared patient for intervention.	___	___	_____
8. Raised bed to comfortable working level.	___	___	_____
9. Arranged for patient privacy.	___	___	_____
10. Positioned patient and waterproof pad appropriately.	___	___	_____
11. Placed refuse container in convenient location away from sterile field.	___	___	_____
12. Set up sterile field.	___	___	_____
13. Donned gown and goggles if appropriate.	___	___	_____
14. Removed dressing and discarded dressing in refuse container.	___	___	_____
15. Assessed status of wound and wound drainage on dressing.	___	___	_____
16. Placed collection basin appropriately.	___	___	_____
17. Removed gloves, washed hands, and donned sterile gloves.	___	___	_____
18. Cleansed area around wound with antiseptic swabs.	___	___	_____
19. Filled irrigating syringe with solution; attached soft catheter if irrigating a deep wound with small opening.	___	___	_____

	S	U	Comments

20. Instilled solution gently into wound, holding syringe approximately 1 inch above wound; if using catheter, gently inserted into wound opening until slight resistance was met, pulled back, and gently instilled solution.

____ ____ _____

21. Allowed solution to flow from clean to dirty area.

____ ____ _____

22. Pinched off catheter during withdrawal from wound.

____ ____ _____

23. Refilled syringe and continued irrigation until solution returned clear.

____ ____ _____

24. Blotted wound edges with sterile gauze.

____ ____ _____

25. Redressed wound if applicable.

____ ____ _____

26. Removed gloves, washed hands, and donned clean gloves.

____ ____ _____

27. Discarded soiled material and contaminated solution appropriately.

____ ____ _____

28. Repositioned patient.

____ ____ _____

29. Removed gloves and washed hands.

____ ____ _____

30. Documented.

____ ____ _____

Performance Checklist
Skill 18–7

REMOVING SUTURES OR STAPLES

	S	U	Comments
1. Obtained equipment.	___	___	_____
2. Referred to medical record, care plan, or Kardex for special interventions.	___	___	_____
3. Introduced self.	___	___	_____
4. Identified patient by identification band.	___	___	_____
5. Explained procedure to patient.	___	___	_____
6. Washed hands and donned clean gloves.	___	___	_____
7. Prepared patient for intervention.	___	___	_____
8. Raised bed to comfortable working level.	___	___	_____
9. Arranged for patient privacy.	___	___	_____
10. Positioned patient.	___	___	_____
11. Placed refuse container in convenient location away from sterile field.	___	___	_____
12. Set up sterile field.	___	___	_____
13. Removed dressing; discarded into plastic refuse bag.	___	___	_____
14. Assessed status of wound and drainage on dressing.	___	___	_____
15. Removed gloves, washed hands, and donned sterile gloves.	___	___	_____
16. Cleansed area with antiseptic swabs, starting from incision outward, one stroke with each swab.	___	___	_____

Removing interrupted sutures

	S	U	Comments
17. Grasped and elevated knotted end of suture with hemostat or forceps.	___	___	_____
18. Cut suture at skin level on opposite side, distal to knot.	___	___	_____

19. Gently removed entire suture with forceps and discarded on sterile gauze, counting as each is removed.

  ____ ____ _____

20. Repeated steps until all sutures have been removed.

  ____ ____ _____

21. Recounted number of sutures removed.

  ____ ____ _____

Removing continuous sutures

22. Cut first suture close to skin on side away from knot.

  ____ ____ _____

23. Removed gently from knotted side with forceps and discarded on sterile gauze, counting as each is removed.

  ____ ____ _____

24. Cut second suture on same side away from knot.

  ____ ____ _____

25. Repeated until all sutures have been removed.

  ____ ____ _____

26. Recounted number of sutures removed.

  ____ ____ _____

Removing staples

27. Placed staple remover under both sides of staple; squeezed handles together and gently removed staple from skin.

  ____ ____ _____

28. Released handles and discarded staple in staple holder, counting as each is removed.

  ____ ____ _____

29. Repeated until all staples have been removed or every other staple has been removed.

  ____ ____ _____

30. Recounted number of staples removed.

  ____ ____ _____

31. Assessed healing status of wound.

  ____ ____ _____

32. Cleansed area with antiseptic swabs.

  ____ ____ _____

33. Applied sterile dressing, steri-stripped wound, or left open to air as applicable.

  ____ ____ _____

34. Removed gloves and washed hands.

  ____ ____ _____

35. Documented.

  ____ ____ _____

Performance Checklist
Skill 19–1

PERFORMING NASOGASTRIC TUBE INSERTION AND TUBE FEEDING

		S	U	Comments
1.	Obtained equipment.	___	___	_____
2.	Referred to medical record, care plan, or Kardex for special interventions.	___	___	_____
3.	Introduced self.	___	___	_____
4.	Identified patient by identification band.	___	___	_____
5.	Explained procedure to patient.	___	___	_____
6.	Washed hands and donned clean gloves.	___	___	_____
7.	Prepared patient for intervention.	___	___	_____
8.	Raised bed to comfortable working level.	___	___	_____
9.	Arranged for patient privacy.	___	___	_____
10.	Assessed condition and patency of nares to determine through which air passed more easily.	___	___	_____
11.	Placed patient in high-Fowler's position and raised bed to comfortable height for patient.	___	___	_____
12.	Stood on dominant side.	___	___	_____
13.	Placed towel or waterproof pad over patient's chest with tissues nearby.	___	___	_____
14.	Determined length of tube to reach stomach.	___	___	_____
15.	Used tape to mark distance for tube to be inserted.	___	___	_____
16.	Cut two pieces of tape, one 3 inches long and $1\frac{1}{2}$ inches long, and tore 3-inch strip halfway down center.	___	___	_____
17.	Lubricated first 3 to 4 inches (7.5 to 10 centimeters) of tube.	___	___	_____
18.	Extended patient's head back toward pillow, held tube about 3 inches from tip and inserted it into nostril, and gently guided it straight back and down along floor of nose.	___	___	_____

	S	**U**	**Comments**

19. Had patient flex head slightly forward as tube was advanced and had patient sip water (if permitted) or swallow as tube was advanced.

20. Withdrew tube slightly if there was excessive gagging and coughing; used flashlight and tongue depressor to assess pharynx.

21. Continued advancing tube until tape mark reached nares.

22. Stopped procedure if patient gasped, become cyanotic, or was unable to speak; let patient relax, relubricated tube, and then reinserted tube.

23. Verified that tube was in stomach.

24. Attached 30-ml syringe to tube; placed stethoscope over epigastric area; while auscultating, injected 10 to 20 ml of air into tube, listening for gurgling sound.

25. Aspirated gastric contents and assessed acidity.

26. Clamped or plugged tube.

27. Had patient close eyes tightly and wiped bridge of nose carefully, avoiding eye area, and allowed 60 seconds to dry.

28. Secured tube to patient's nose with tape and to gown with rubber band and safety pin.

29. Pressed wide part of 3-inch tape over bridge of nose lengthwise.

30. Left head of bed elevated for tube feeding and made patient comfortable.

Administering enteral feedings

31. Assessed placement of tube before instilling liquid, aspirated gastric contents and measured for residual, and reinstilled contents according to agency policy.

Intermittent bolus feeding

32. Clamped end of feeding tube.

33. Attached syringe to end of tube.

34. Filled syringe with formula and raised syringe 18 inches above port of entry.

35. Unclamped tubing and allowed syringe to empty gradually to just above connection; refilled repeatedly until prescribed volume had been instilled.

PERFORMING NASOGASTRIC TUBE INSERTION AND TUBE FEEDING (Continued)

	S	U	Comments

Continuous feeding

36. Filled bag and tubing with formula as prescribed and attached to clamped nasogastric tube.

37. Connected infusion pump and set rate; removed clamp from connection and allowed formula to be delivered.

38. Administered additional water as prescribed or according to agency policy.

39. Clamped or plugged feeding tube when not being used.

40. Removed gloves and washed hands.

41. Documented.

Performance Checklist
Skill 19–2

PERFORMING GASTROSTOMY AND JEJUNOSTOMY TUBE CARE

	S	U	Comments
1. Obtained equipment.			
2. Referred to medical record, care plan, or Kardex for special interventions.			
3. Introduced self.			
4. Identified patient by identification band.			
5. Explained procedure to patient.			
6. Washed hands and donned clean gloves.			
7. Prepared patient for intervention.			
8. Raised bed to comfortable level.			
9. Arranged for patient privacy.			
10. Inspected skin around gastrostomy tube for color, breaks, and presence of drainage, odor, and swelling; measured length of tube.			
11. Palpated abdomen and listened for bowel sounds.			
12. Assisted patient to comfortable position that allowed access to dressing.			
13. Placed an open, cuffed plastic bag within easy reach.			
14. Loosened tape by pulling toward dressing.			
15. Removed dressing and assessed drainage.			
16. Discarded dressing in plastic bag.			
17. Measured length of tube.			
18. Cleansed skin with soap and water and dried well.			
19. Replaced dressing and tape using sterile technique.			

	S	U	Comments

20. Weighed patient and discussed frequency, amount, and type of feedings. ____ ____ _____

21. Provided mouth care if necessary. ____ ____ _____

22. Removed gloves and washed hands. ____ ____ _____

23. Documented. ____ ____ _____

Performance Checklist
Skill 19–3

PERFORMING GASTRIC LAVAGE OR IRRIGATION

	S	U	Comments
1. Obtained equipment.			
2. Referred to medical record, care plan, or Kardex for special interventions.			
3. Introduced self.			
4. Identified patient by identification band.			
5. Explained procedure to patient.			
6. Washed hands and donned clean gloves.			
7. Prepared patient for intervention.			
8. Raised bed to comfortable working level.			
9. Arranged for patient privacy.			
10. Assessed functioning of suction apparatus and suction tubing.			
11. Assessed abdomen.			
12. Placed patient in semi-Fowler's position.			
13. Disconnected nasogastric tubing and placed suction tubing on waterproof pad or towel.			
14. Verified that tube was in stomach.			
15. Attached syringe to tube and aspirated gastric contents.			
16. Placed stethoscope over epigastric area if no gastric contents are aspirated and auscultated while injecting 20 to 30 ml of air into tube.			
17. Poured normal saline into container and drew 30 ml (or amount ordered) into irrigating syringe.			
18. Placed syringe into nasogastric tube while pinching between index finger and thumb and kept syringe in upright position; gently instilled solution without using force.			
19. Changed patient's position and repeated steps if no resistance met.			

	S	U	Comments

20. Withdrew fluid into syringe and measured; continued irrigating with appropriate amount of normal saline or until purpose of treatment was accomplished. ____ ____ _____

21. Reclamped or plugged nasogastric tube or reconnected it to suction tubing. ____ ____ _____

22. Assessed and recorded amount of saline instilled and withdrawn. ____ ____ _____

23. Removed gloves and washed hands. ____ ____ _____

24. Documented. ____ ____ _____

Performance Checklist
Skill 19–4

PERFORMING GASTRIC SUCTIONING

		S	U	Comments
1.	Obtained equipment.	___	___	_____
2.	Referred to medical record, care plan, or Kardex for special interventions.	___	___	_____
3.	Introduced self.	___	___	_____
4.	Identified patient by identification band.	___	___	_____
5.	Explained procedure to patient.	___	___	_____
6.	Washed hands and donned clean gloves.	___	___	_____
7.	Prepared patient for intervention.	___	___	_____
8.	Raised bed to comfortable working level.	___	___	_____
9.	Arranged for patient privacy.	___	___	_____
10.	Assessed patient's oral and nasal cavities.	___	___	_____
11.	Assessed patient's abdomen for bowel sounds and amount of distention.	___	___	_____
12.	Assessed suction apparatus according to type.	___	___	_____
13.	Assessed for kinks and ensured patient was not lying on tube.	___	___	_____
14.	Ensured that nasogastric tube was pinned to patient's gown with enough slack to allow movement.	___	___	_____
15.	Ensured that drainage was moving through tubing to drainage-collection bottle.	___	___	_____
16.	Listened at opening of blue air vent, making certain that vent was pointing upward for Salem sump tube.	___	___	_____
17.	Estimated amount of drainage in bottle and emptied it if full and at end of shift.	___	___	_____
18.	Removed gloves and washed hands.	___	___	_____
19.	Documented.	___	___	_____

Performance Checklist
Skill 19–5

REMOVING A NASOGASTRIC TUBE

	S	U	Comments
1. Obtained equipment.	____	____	_____
2. Referred to medical record, care plan, or Kardex for special interventions.	____	____	_____
3. Introduced self.	____	____	_____
4. Identified patient by identification band.	____	____	_____
5. Explained procedure to patient.	____	____	_____
6. Washed hands and donned clean gloves.	____	____	_____
7. Prepared patient for intervention.	____	____	_____
8. Raised bed to comfortable working level.	____	____	_____
9. Arranged for patient privacy.	____	____	_____
10. Assessed nose and oral cavity.	____	____	_____
11. Assessed patient's abdomen.	____	____	_____
12. Turned off suction and disconnected tubing if tube was attached to suction.	____	____	_____
13. Removed tape from nose and pin from gown.	____	____	_____
14. Placed towel or waterproof pad across patient's chest and provided facial tissues.	____	____	_____
15. Pinched tube with fingers or clamped; quickly and smoothly removed tube while patient holds breath.	____	____	_____
16. Placed tube in plastic bag.	____	____	_____
17. Provided oronasal care and made sure patient was comfortable.	____	____	_____
18. Disposed of tube and equipment and measured drainage.	____	____	_____
19. Removed gloves and washed hands.	____	____	_____
20. Documented.	____	____	_____

Performance Checklist
Skill 20–1

POSITIONING, MOVING, AND LIFTING THE PATIENT

	S	U	Comments
1. Obtained equipment.	___	___	_____
2. Referred to medical record, care plan, or Kardex for special interventions.	___	___	_____
3. Introduced self.	___	___	_____
4. Identified patient by identification band.	___	___	_____
5. Explained procedure to patient.	___	___	_____
6. Washed hands and donned clean gloves.	___	___	_____
7. Prepared patient for intervention.	___	___	_____
8. Raised bed to comfortable working level.	___	___	_____
9. Arranged for patient privacy.	___	___	_____

Positioning patient

Dorsal (supine)

	S	U	Comments
10. Moved patient and mattress to head of bed and removed pillow.	___	___	_____
11. Lowered head of bed unless contraindicated.	___	___	_____
12. Turned patient onto back.	___	___	_____
13. Replaced pillow.	___	___	_____
14. Removed gloves and washed hands.	___	___	_____

Dorsal-recumbent

	S	U	Comments
15. Moved patient and mattress to head of bed and removed pillow.	___	___	_____
16. Lowered head of bed unless contraindicated.	___	___	_____
17. Turned patient onto back.	___	___	_____
18. Assisted patient to raise legs and bend knees and allowed legs to relax.	___	___	_____
19. Replaced pillow.	___	___	_____
20. Removed gloves and washed hands.	___	___	_____

	S	U	Comments

Fowler's

21. Moved patient and mattress to head of bed and removed pillow.

22. Raised head of bed to 45 to 60 degrees.

23. Replaced pillow.

24. Raised foot of bed no more than 15 degrees.

25. Removed gloves and washed hands.

Knee-chest

26. Turned patient onto abdomen.

27. Assisted patient to kneeling position; arms and head should rest on pillow while upper chest rests on bed.

28. Removed gloves and washed hands.

Lithotomy

29. Requested patient to move buttocks to edge of examining table.

30. Lifted both legs, had patient bend knees, and placed feet in stirrups at the same time.

31. Draped patient.

32. Removed gloves and washed hands.

Orthopneic

33. Elevated head of bed to 90 degrees.

34. Placed pillow between patient's back and mattress.

35. Placed pillow on overbed table and assisted patient to lean over, placing head on pillow.

36. Removed gloves and washed hands.

Prone

37. Assisted patient onto abdomen with face to one side.

38. Flexed arms toward head.

39. Removed gloves and washed hands.

Semi-Fowler's

40. Moved patient and mattress to head of bed and removed pillow.

41. Raised head of bed to about 30 degrees.

42. Replaced pillow.

43. Slightly raised foot of bed.

44. Removed gloves and washed hands

**Performance Checklist
Skill 20–1**

POSITIONING, MOVING, AND LIFTING THE PATIENT
(Continued)

	S	U	Comments

Sims'

45. Moved patient and mattress to head of bed and removed pillow.

46. Turned patient to right side.

47. Assisted patient to draw left knee and thigh up near abdomen.

48. Placed patient's right arm along the back.

49. Allowed patient to lean forward to rest on chest.

50. Removed gloves and washed hands.

Trendelenburg's

51. Placed patient's head lower than body, with body and legs elevated on an incline.

52. Removed gloves and washed hands.

Moving the patient

53. Obtained equipment.

Lifting and moving patient up in bed

54. Placed patient supine with head flat.

55. Faced side of bed and provided base of support.

56. Placed one arm under axilla (two nurses) and opposite arm under shoulder and neck.

57. Requested patient flex knees and push up with feet on count of 3 while assisting.

58. On count of 3, each nurse pulled patient up to head of bed with minimum friction.

59. One nurse may perform procedure if patient able to move freely.

	S	U	Comments

Turning the patient

60. Stood with feet slightly apart and flexed knees.

_____ _____ _____

61. Placed arm under patient's neck and shoulders and opposite arm under patient's waist.

_____ _____ _____

62. Pulled patient toward self.

_____ _____ _____

63. Turned patient on side facing self and raised side rail.

_____ _____ _____

64. Flexed one leg over other.

_____ _____ _____

65. Aligned shoulders.

_____ _____ _____

66. Supported back with pillows if necessary.

_____ _____ _____

67. Assessed body alignment by standing at foot of bed looking straight at patient.

_____ _____ _____

Logrolling patient

68. Three nurses stood side by side of bed.

_____ _____ _____

69. One nurse placed arms under legs; second nurse placed arms under buttocks; third nurse placed arms under chest, shoulders, and neck.

_____ _____ _____

70. Nurse nearest head of patient gave prearranged signal and turned patient at exact same time.

_____ _____ _____

71. Made patient comfortable.

_____ _____ _____

72. Removed gloves and washed hands.

_____ _____ _____

Transferring patient from bed to straight chair and wheelchair

73. Lowered bed to lowest position.

_____ _____ _____

74. Raised head of bed.

_____ _____ _____

75. Supported patient's shoulder and helped patient swing legs around and off bed; performed all in one motion.

_____ _____ _____

76. Assisted patient to don robe and slippers.

_____ _____ _____

77. Had chair preplaced beside bed, with seat facing head of bed.

_____ _____ _____

78. Locked wheelchair.

_____ _____ _____

79. Placed straight chair against wall or had another nurse hold chair.

_____ _____ _____

80. Stood directly in front of patient and placed hands under patient's axillae.

_____ _____ _____

81. Assisted patient to stand and swing around with back toward seat of chair.

_____ _____ _____

**Performance Checklist
Skill 20–1**

POSITIONING, MOVING, AND LIFTING THE PATIENT
(Continued)

	S	U	Comments

82. Assisted patient to sit down as nurse bent knees to assist process.

83. Applied blanket to legs if needed.

84. Removed gloves and washed hands.

Using the lift for moving patient

85. Secured appropriate number of personnel to assist.

86. Placed chair near bed.

87. Raised bed to maximum height.

88. Placed canvas seat evenly under patient.

89. Slid horseshoe-shaped bar under bed on side.

90. Lowered horizontal bar to level of sling by releasing hydraulic valve and locked valve.

91. Fastened hook on chain to holes in sling.

92. Raised head of bed.

93. Folded patient's arms over chest.

94. Pumped life-handle until patient was raised off bed.

95. With steering handle, pulled lift off bed and down to chair.

96. Released valve *slowly* to left and lowered patient to chair.

97. Closed off valve and released straps.

98. Removed straps and lift.

99. Removed gloves and washed hands.

100. Documented.

Performance Checklist
Skill 20–2

PERFORMING PASSIVE RANGE-OF-MOTION EXERCISES

	S	U	Comments
1. Obtained equipment.	____	____	_____
2. Referred to medical record, care plan, or Kardex for special interventions.	____	____	_____
3. Introduced self.	____	____	_____
4. Identified patient by identification band.	____	____	_____
5. Explained procedure to patient.	____	____	_____
6. Washed hands and donned clean gloves.	____	____	_____
7. Prepared patient for intervention.	____	____	_____
8. Raised bed to comfortable working level.	____	____	_____
9. Arranged for patient privacy.	____	____	_____
10. Assisted patient by putting each joint through full range of motion.	____	____	_____
11. Adjusted bed linen.	____	____	_____
12. Removed gloves and washed hands.	____	____	_____
13. Documented.	____	____	_____

**Performance Checklist
Skill 21–1**

CARING FOR A PRESSURE ULCER

	S	U	Comments
1. Obtained equipment.	___	___	_____
2. Referred to medical record, care plan, or Kardex for special interventions.	___	___	_____
3. Introduced self.	___	___	_____
4. Identified patient by identification band.	___	___	_____
5. Explained procedure to patient.	___	___	_____
6. Washed hands and donned clean gloves.	___	___	_____
7. Prepared patient for intervention.	___	___	_____
8. Raised bed to comfortable working level.	___	___	_____
9. Arranged for patient privacy.	___	___	_____
10. Assessed pressure ulcer.	___	___	_____
11. Assessed for high risk for developing pressure ulcer.	___	___	_____
12. Removed ulcer dressing and assessed drainage and healing.	___	___	_____
13. Measured pressure for length, width, and depth.	___	___	_____
14. Cleansed ulcer with appropriate agent and irrigated if deep ulcer.	___	___	_____
15. Applied medication as prescribed.	___	___	_____
16. Applied sterile dressing.	___	___	_____
17. Removed gloves and washed hands.	___	___	_____
18. Documented.	___	___	_____

Performance Checklist
Skill 22–1

APPLYING RESTRAINTS

	S	U	Comments
1. Obtained equipment.	___	___	_____
2. Referred to medical record, care plan, or Kardex for special interventions.	___	___	_____
3. Introduced self.	___	___	_____
4. Identified patient by identification band.	___	___	_____
5. Explained procedure to patient.	___	___	_____
6. Washed hands and donned clean gloves according to agency policy, OSHA, and CDC guidelines.	___	___	_____
7. Prepared patient for intervention.	___	___	_____
8. Raised bed to comfortable working level.	___	___	_____
9. Arranged for patient privacy.	___	___	_____
10. Assessed patient's potential for injury.	___	___	_____
11. Wrist or ankle (extremity restraint):			
• Made clove hitch if Kerlix was used.	___	___	_____
• Placed gauze or padding around extremity.	___	___	_____
• Slipped wrist or ankle through loops directly over padding.	___	___	_____
• Wrapped padded portion of restraint around affected extremity, threaded through slit in restraint, and fastened to second tie with secure knot.	___	___	_____
• Tied ends of restraint in a bow (not to side rails).	___	___	_____
• Left as much slack as possible.	___	___	_____
• Palpated pulses below restraint.	___	___	_____
• Monitored skin for irritation.	___	___	_____
• Assessed circulation to extremity distal to restraint at least every 2 hours.	___	___	_____

168

	S	U	Comments

12. Elbow Restraint:

- Placed restraint and piece of fabric with slots for insertion of tongue depressors (blades) to keep elbow straight over elbow. _____ _____ _____

- Wrapped restraint snugly, tying restraints at top. _____ _____ _____

- Monitored position of restraint, circulation, and skin condition frequently. _____ _____ _____

13. Vest (jacket or chest) restraint:

- Applied restraint over patient's gown. _____ _____ _____

- Placed vest on with V opening in front or fastened with velcro and zipper. _____ _____ _____

- Pulled tie at end of vest flap across chest and slipped tie through slit on opposite side of vest. _____ _____ _____

- Wrapped other end of flap across patient and tied straps in bow to frame of bed or behind wheelchair where patient cannot untie. _____ _____ _____

- Made room for fist in space between vest and patient. _____ _____ _____

- Monitored respiratory status. _____ _____ _____

14. Removed restraints every 2 hours according to agency policy and patient need and avoided leaving patient alone during this time. _____ _____ _____

15. Washed, rinsed, dried, and massaged skin areas with lotion. _____ _____ _____

16. Performed range-of-motion exercises when restraints were removed. _____ _____ _____

17. Removed gloves and washed hands. _____ _____ _____

18. Documented. _____ _____ _____

**Performance Checklist
Skill 22–2**

CARING FOR VICTIMS OF ACCIDENTAL POISONING

	S	U	Comments
1. Obtained equipment.	____	____	_____
2. Referred to medical record, care plan, or Kardex for special interventions.	____	____	_____
3. Introduced self.	____	____	_____
4. Identified patient by identification band.	____	____	_____
5. Explained procedure to patient.	____	____	_____
6. Washed hands and donned clean gloves.	____	____	_____
7. Prepared patient for intervention.	____	____	_____
8. Raised bed to comfortable working level.	____	____	_____
9. Arranged for patient privacy.	____	____	_____
10. Notified poison control center or followed agency protocols.	____	____	_____
11. If instructed, used ipecac to induce vomiting, following dosage instructions, and provided adequate fluids.	____	____	_____
• Made certain gag reflex was intact.	____	____	_____
• If instructed, saved emesis.	____	____	_____
• Placed patient's head to one side.	____	____	_____
12. Did not induce vomiting if poisoning related to following substances: household cleaners, lye, furniture polish, grease, or petroleum products.	____	____	_____
13. Did not induce vomiting in an unconscious patient.	____	____	_____
14. Continued to monitor vital signs and patient's response to treatment.	____	____	_____
15. Removed gloves and washed hands.	____	____	_____
16. Documented.	____	____	_____

Performance Checklist
Skill 23–1

MAKING A BED

	S	U	Comments
1. Obtained equipment.	___	___	_____
2. Referred to medical record, care plan, or Kardex for special interventions.	___	___	_____
3. Introduced self.	___	___	_____
4. Identified patient by identification band.	___	___	_____
5. Explained procedure to patient.	___	___	_____
6. Washed hands and donned clean gloves.	___	___	_____
7. Prepared patient for intervention.	___	___	_____
8. Raised bed to comfortable working level.	___	___	_____
9. Arranged for patient privacy.	___	___	_____
10. Assessed for urinary or fecal incontinence.	___	___	_____
11. Assessed for personal items in bed.	___	___	_____

Unoccupied bed

	S	U	Comments
12. Placed linens in order of use on seat of straight chair.	___	___	_____
13. Placed laundry bag over back of straight chair.	___	___	_____
14. Removed pillow case from pillow and placed pillow under stack of linen.	___	___	_____
15. Loosened bed linens from under mattress on side of bed where nurse was standing.	___	___	_____
16. Removed and folded bedspread and placed on pillow unless soiled.	___	___	_____
17. Folded bed sheets inward toward middle of bed.	___	___	_____
18. Placed bundle of bed linens into laundry bag.	___	___	_____
19. Straightened and moved mattress to head of bed.	___	___	_____
20. Laid bottom sheet on mattress and unfolded from top to foot of bed; placed soiled linens into laundry bag.	___	___	_____

	S	U	Comments

21. Placed bottom sheet on bed, hem-side down at edge of foot of mattress and excess sheet at head of bed.

22. Tucked bottom sheet in at head of bed while standing in front of work.

23. Mitered corner at head of bed and tucked sheet under one third of mattress.

24. Placed top sheet over bed with raw edge of hem facing up and excess sheet at foot of bed.

25. Completed one side of bed before walking to opposite side.

26. Loosened bed linen under mattress on opposite side of bed.

27. Completed opposite side of bed, mitering corner at head of bed and pulling bottom sheet tight and removing all wrinkles.

28. Placed bedspread on bed about 2 inches down from hem of sheet at head of bed; tucked in tightly at foot and mitered sheet corner and spread together; bedspread should hang below sheet on side of bed toward door.

29. Turned sheet down over bedspread about 2 inches.

30. Placed clean pillow case on pillow.

31. Reviewed work to ensure neat and finished look to bed.

Open bed
(linens fanfolded at foot for easy patient access)

32. Fanfolded top sheet and bedspread to foot of bed.

33. Replaced pillow with open end away from door to room and seam edge away from where patient's head will rest.

34. Removed pillow case from pillow and placed it in laundry bag.

35. Placed pillow under bed linen on straight chair.

36. Turned patient toward opposite side of bed with side rail in up position.

37. Straightened mattress and moved to head of bed.

38. Loosened bed linens from under mattress on side of bed where nurse is standing.

39. Removed and folded bedspread and placed on pillow unless soiled.

Performance Checklist
Skill 23–1

MAKING A BED (Continued)

	S	U	Comments

40. Folded soiled sheets inward toward middle of bed and gently pushed them under patient's back.

41. Laid bottom sheet on mattress and unfolded from top to foot of bed.

42. Placed bottom sheet on bed, hem-side down at edge of foot of mattress with excess sheet at head of bed.

43. Tucked bottom sheet in at head of bed while standing in front of work (applied drawsheet now if policy dictated).

44. Mitered corner at head of bed; then tucked sheet under one third of mattress; pushed soiled linens upward toward patient and gently fanfolded under patient.

45. Placed top sheet over bed with raw edge if hem facing up and with excess at foot of bed.

46. Completed one side of bed before walking to opposite side; moved to opposite side of bed.

47. Loosened bed linen under mattress on opposite side of bed.

48. Completed opposite side of bed, mitering corner at head of bed and pulling bottom sheet tight and removing all wrinkles.

49. Placed bedspread on bed about 2 inches down from hem of sheet at head of bed; tucked in tightly at foot and mitered sheet corner and bedspread together; bedspread should hang below sheet on side of bed toward door.

50. Turned sheet hem down over bedspread about 2 inches on both sides of bed.

51. Placed clean pillow case on pillow.

52. Review work to ensure a neat and finished look to bed.

53. Made a toe pleat for patient.

	S	U	Comments

Orthopedic bed
(specially designed bed for patient in traction)

54. Placed bottom sheet at head of bed and tucked and pulled sheet down under patient's shoulders, waist, and legs to foot of bed.

55. Tucked bottom sheet and mitered corners or allowed top sheet to hang loose at foot if traction apparatus was attached to foot of bed, footboard was used, or bed cradle was in place on top of bed.

56. Kept patient warm, especially feet when bed sheet hung loose from bed.

57. Disposed of dirty linens.

58. Straightened rest of room.

59. Removed gloves and washed hands.

Performance Checklist
Skill 23–2

BATHING A PATIENT

		S	U	Comments
1.	Obtained equipment.			
2.	Referred to medical record, care plan, or Kardex for special interventions.			
3.	Introduced self.			
4.	Identified patient by identification band.			
5.	Explained procedure to patient.			
6.	Washed hands and donned clean gloves.			
7.	Prepared patient for intervention.			
8.	Raised bed to comfortable working level.			
9.	Arranged for patient privacy.			
10.	Assessed patient's skin integrity.			
11.	Assessed patient's likes and dislikes regarding bathing depending on condition.			

Bed Bath

		S	U	Comments
12.	Offered bedpan or urinal and allowed patient to wash hands afterward.			
13.	Provided oral hygiene.			
14.	Removed pillow unless contraindicated and placed pillow case in laundry bag.			
15.	Replaced top linen with bath blanket, placing soiled linens in laundry bag.			
16.	Removed patient's bedclothes and jewelry, securing their safety.			
17.	Filled bath basin one-third to one-half full with hot water.			
18.	Moved patient in supine position to side of bed toward nurse.			
19.	Folded cloth to form mitt and washed eyes with water only from inner aspect to outer aspect.			

	S	U	Comments

20. Washed, rinsed, and dried face, neck, and ears; used towel to drape area bathed.

21. Washed, rinsed, and dried first one arm and then the other using long, firm strokes; allowed patient to place both hands in basin to wash and soak or had them washed with soap and water, rinsed, and dried.

22. Washed, rinsed, and dried chest and breasts without exposure.

23. Washed, rinsed, and dried abdomen, providing attention to umbilicus, using long, firm strokes.

24. Changed bath water and prepared as before.

25. Washed, rinsed, and dried one leg; soaked and washed foot in basin by flexing knee and placing foot in bath basin, protecting heel from causing pressure on heel; kept patient adequately draped to prevent genital area from being exposed; assessed patient regarding being ticklish to prevent foot from spilling water from basin onto bed, patient, and nurse.

26. Repeated above steps on opposite leg and foot.

27. Changed bath water and prepared as before.

28. Washed, rinsed, and dried back and buttocks using long, firm strokes.

29. Administered 3 to 5 minute backrub using lotion warmed in hands and rubbed back and buttocks with circular motions unless contraindicated.

30. Washed, rinsed, and dried genitals or allowed patient to finish bath if able.

31. Applied clean bedclothes.

32. Emptied and cleaned bath basin.

33. Combed hair, shaved male patient, and arranged for makeup for female; assisted as necessary with grooming.

34. Turned patient toward opposite side of bed with side rail in up position.

35. Moved mattress up to head of bed.

36. Made occupied bed.

Partial Bath

37. Assisted with bathing parts of body unable to reach; assisted with oral hygiene.

**Performance Checklist
Skill 23–2**

BATHING A PATIENT (Continued)

	S	U	Comments

38. Administered 3 to 5 minute backrub using lotion warmed in hands and rubbed back and buttocks using circular motions unless contraindicated. _____ _____ _____

39. Made open bed. _____ _____ _____

Shower or Tub Bath

40. Assisted patient as necessary to tub or shower room. _____ _____ _____

41. Arranged for oral hygiene. _____ _____ _____

42. Made open bed. _____ _____ _____

Sitz Bath

43. Arranged for oral hygiene. _____ _____ _____

44. Ran appropriate amount and temperature of water in tub; ran water to come just to patient's hips. _____ _____ _____

45. Assisted patient into tub; arranged more assistance if necessary. _____ _____ _____

46. Timed bath for 15 to 20 minutes depending on if first time to take bath. _____ _____ _____

47. Assisted patient from tub, arranged more assistance if necessary, and patted skin dry. _____ _____ _____

48. Assisted patient back to room. _____ _____ _____

49. Assisted patient to chair if able and made open bed. _____ _____ _____

Tepid Sponge Bath

50. Assessed body temperature before sponging. _____ _____ _____

51. Applied bath blanket over patient. _____ _____ _____

52. Placed warm, wet cloth on face and warmed towels over body for 20 to 30 minutes. _____ _____ _____

53. Reassessed body temperature. _____ _____ _____

	S	**U**	**Comments**

54. Continued sponging at 15-minute intervals or until temperature reduced to normal or until reduced; assessed condition of patient throughout procedure for complications.   ___ ___ _____

55. Dried patient gently; dressed and provided warmth.   ___ ___ _____

56. Remade bed if necessary.   ___ ___ _____

57. Removed gloves and washed hands.   ___ ___ _____

58. Documented.   ___ ___ _____

Performance Checklist
Skill 23–3

ASSISTING WITH ORAL HYGIENE

	S	U	Comments
1. Obtained equipment.	___	___	_____
2. Referred to medical record, care plan, or Kardex for special interventions.	___	___	_____
3. Introduced self.	___	___	_____
4. Identified patient by identification band.	___	___	_____
5. Explained procedure to patient.	___	___	_____
6. Washed hands and donned clean gloves.	___	___	_____
7. Prepared patient for intervention.	___	___	_____
8. Raised bed to comfortable working level.	___	___	_____
9. Arranged for patient privacy.	___	___	_____
10. Assessed patient's ability to perform oral hygiene.	___	___	_____
11. Arranged towel over patient's chest.	___	___	_____
12. Wet toothbrush, applied toothpaste, and allowed patient to brush teeth and gums at 45-degree angle.	___	___	_____
13. Provided patient with water for rinsing mouth.	___	___	_____
14. Provided dental floss.	___	___	_____
15. Allowed patient to rinse again.	___	___	_____
16. Cleaned and replaced articles.	___	___	_____
17. Removed gloves and washed hands.	___	___	_____
18. Documented.	___	___	_____

**Performance Checklist
Skill 23–4**

CARING FOR THE HAIR

	S	U	Comments
1. Obtained equipment			
2. Referred to medical record, care plan, or Kardex for special interventions.			
3. Introduced self.			
4. Identified patient by identification band.			
5. Explained procedure to patient.			
6. Washed hands and donned clean gloves.			
7. Prepared patient for intervention.			
8. Raised bed to comfortable working level.			
9. Arranged for patient privacy.			
10. Assessed patient's hair regarding cleanliness, texture, distribution, scalp lesions, and infestation.			
11. Assessed type of care patient uses for hair and if it is appropriate.			
12. Placed towel around shoulders if patient is able to sit or under head, if not.			
13. Combed or assisted in combing patient's hair by sections.			
14. Removed towel by folding it away from gown.			
15. Removed gloves and washed hands.			
16. Ensured that combing hair was included in bath and AM care.			

**Performance Checklist
Skill 23–5**

CARING FOR THE HANDS, FEET, AND NAILS

	S	U	Comments
1. Obtained equipment.	___	___	_____
2. Referred to medical record, care plan, or Kardex for special interventions.	___	___	_____
3. Introduced self.	___	___	_____
4. Identified patient by identification band.	___	___	_____
5. Explained procedure to patient.	___	___	_____
6. Washed hands and donned clean gloves.	___	___	_____
7. Prepared patient for intervention.	___	___	_____
8. Raised bed to comfortable working level.	___	___	_____
9. Arranged for patient privacy.	___	___	_____
10. Assessed color and sensation of fingers, nails, and feet.	___	___	_____
11. Assessed for breaks in skin or cracking of fingers, nails, feet, and toes.	___	___	_____
12. Assessed patient's knowledge of care of fingers, nails, feet, and toes.	___	___	_____

Care of Feet and Toenails

13. Filled basin one-half full of warm water.	___	___	_____
14. Assisted patient in placing feet in warm water to soak.	___	___	_____
15. After soaking nails and feet for 10 to 15 minutes, dried feet by patting and carefully cleaned nails with orange stick; clipped nails straight across or filed with nail file unless contraindicated.	___	___	_____

Care of Hands and Fingernails

16. Soaked hands for 10 to 15 minutes in warm water.	___	___	_____

	S	U	Comments

17. Dried hands by patting and carefully cleaned nails with orange stick; clipped nails straight across or filed with nail file unless contraindicated. _____ _____ _____

18. Removed gloves and washed hands. _____ _____ _____

19. Documented special care of hands, feet, and nails. (Routine care usually is not documented.) _____ _____ _____

Performance Checklist
Skill 23–6

SHAVING THE MALE PATIENT

		S	U	Comments
1.	Obtained equipment.	___	___	_____
2.	Referred to medical record, care plan, or Kardex for special interventions.	___	___	_____
3.	Introduced self.	___	___	_____
4.	Identified patient by identification band.	___	___	_____
5.	Explained procedure to patient.	___	___	_____
6.	Washed hands and donned clean gloves.	___	___	_____
7.	Prepared patient for intervention.	___	___	_____
8.	Raised bed to comfortable working level.	___	___	_____
9.	Arranged for patient privacy.	___	___	_____
10.	Assessed patient for bleeding problems.	___	___	_____
11.	Assessed patient's emotional status.	___	___	_____
12.	Placed patient in semi-Fowler's position unless contraindicated.	___	___	_____
13.	Placed very warm wet washcloth over patient's face, avoiding burning.	___	___	_____
14.	Applied shaving cream to face.	___	___	_____
15.	Began shaving from ear downward to near mouth; rinsed razor.	___	___	_____
16.	Continued this step until face was completely shaved, rinsing razor often.	___	___	_____
17.	Shaved from under nose downward to shave upper lip; rinsed razor.	___	___	_____
18.	Rinsed face and dried by patting.	___	___	_____
19.	Applied aftershave lotion if patient desired.	___	___	_____
20.	Repositioned patient as required.	___	___	_____
21.	Removed gloves and washed hands.	___	___	_____
22.	Documented according to agency policy (considered part of bath process in some agencies).	___	___	_____

Performance Checklist
Skill 23–7

ASSISTING WITH THE BEDPAN AND URINAL

	S	U	Comments
1. Obtained equipment.	___	___	_____
2. Referred to medical record, care plan, or Kardex for special interventions.	___	___	_____
3. Introduced self.	___	___	_____
4. Identified patient by identification band.	___	___	_____
5. Explained procedure to patient.	___	___	_____
6. Washed hands and donned clean gloves.	___	___	_____
7. Prepared patient for intervention.	___	___	_____
8. Raised bed to comfortable working level.	___	___	_____
9. Arranged for patient privacy.	___	___	_____
10. Assessed patient's need for assistance.	___	___	_____
11. Placed protector under patient.	___	___	_____
12. Warmed metal bedpan or metal urinal under running warm water.	___	___	_____

For Patient Unable to Assist Self on Bedpan

	S	U	Comments
13. Turned patient away from nurse toward opposite side rail, moving linens out of way.	___	___	_____
14. Fitted bedpan to patient's buttocks.	___	___	_____
15. Assisted patient to turn over with bedpan while nurse held bedpan securely, and raised head of bed to 30 degrees.	___	___	_____
16. Arranged toilet tissue and call light within easy reach.	___	___	_____
17. Allowed patient time to eliminate or remained in room if condition warranted, allowing as much privacy as possible.	___	___	_____
18. Assisted in cleaning perineal area if needed.	___	___	_____
19. Removed bedpan as it was applied.	___	___	_____

	S	**U**	**Comments**

For Patient Able to Assist Self on Bedpan

20. Moved bed linens out of way.

21. Asked patient to raise buttocks off bed while nurse supported back.

22. Slid warmed bedpan under patient's buttocks.

23. Asked patient to sit on bedpan while nurse adjusted comfort level.

24. Rolled head of bed up to tolerance, arranged toilet tissue, and placed call light within easy reach of patient.

25. Moved linens away from genital area without exposure.

26. Lifted penis gently, and placed in urinal if patient unable to do so. (If patient was able, allowed patient to handle urinal for voiding.)

27. Replaced bed linens over patient.

28. Allowed patient to void unless needing assistance.

29. Removed urinal and assisted patient as needed.

30. Emptied urinal in graduate and measured urine; cleansed and replaced urinal.

31. Removed gloves and washed hands.

32. Documented.

MEASURING AND RECORDING FLUID INTAKE AND OUTPUT

	S	U	Comments
1. Obtained equipment.	___	___	_____
2. Referred to medical record, care plan, or Kardex for special interventions.	___	___	_____
3. Introduced self.	___	___	_____
4. Identified patient by identification band.	___	___	_____
5. Explained procedure to patient.	___	___	_____
6. Washed hands and donned clean gloves.	___	___	_____
7. Prepared patient for intervention.	___	___	_____
8. Raised bed to comfortable working level.	___	___	_____
9. Arranged for patient privacy.	___	___	_____
10. Measured and recorded all fluids taken orally, including tube feedings, parenteral fluids, blood components, total parenteral nutrition, and foods that melt at room temperature.	___	___	_____
11. Informed patient not to empty any body excreta but to contact nurse as needed.	___	___	_____
12. Instructed patient to inform nurse of all oral intake or record amounts on intake and output form.	___	___	_____
13. Measured and recorded drainage from Foley catheter drainage system, nasogastric suction, surgical wound receptacles, emesis, and diarrhea stools every 8 hours.	___	___	_____
14. Removed gloves and washed hands.	___	___	_____
15. Documented.	___	___	_____

SERVING FOOD AND ASSISTING WITH FEEDING A PATIENT

	S	U	Comments
1. Obtained equipment.	____	____	_____
2. Referred to medical record, care plan, or Kardex for special interventions.	____	____	_____
3. Introduced self.	____	____	_____
4. Identified patient by identification band.	____	____	_____
5. Offered pain medication or other medication if indicated.	____	____	_____
6. Washed hands and donned clean gloves.	____	____	_____
7. Offered bedpan or urinal if needed.	____	____	_____
8. Prepared patient for intervention.	____	____	_____
9. Raised bed to comfortable working level.	____	____	_____
10. Arranged for patient privacy.	____	____	_____
11. Assisted with oral hygiene if needed.	____	____	_____
12. Provided water, soap, and towel for patient's hands and face if needed.	____	____	_____
13. Cleared off over-bed table.	____	____	_____
14. Obtained food tray and assessed for correct diet.	____	____	_____
15. Assisted with food preparation as needed.	____	____	_____
16. Removed tray when patient was finished.	____	____	_____
17. Raised side rail if needed.	____	____	_____
18. Assessed and recorded amount of food eaten.	____	____	_____

Assisting with Feeding Patient

	S	U	Comments
19. Assessed patient's ability to self-feed and assisted if necessary.	____	____	_____
20. Offered medication if needed.	____	____	_____
21. Offered bedpan or urinal if needed.	____	____	_____
22. Assisted with oral hygiene if needed.	____	____	_____

	S	U	Comments

23. Washed patient's face and hands as needed. ____ ____ _____

24. Cleared off over-bed table. ____ ____ _____

25. Obtained food tray and assessed for correct diet. ____ ____ _____

26. Placed napkin under patient's chin. ____ ____ _____

27. Buttered bread and cut meat if needed, opened liquid cartons, poured hot liquids, prepared tea or coffee as patient desired, and provided drinking straw for liquids. ____ ____ _____

28. Encouraged patient to eat without assistance. ____ ____ _____

29. Gave solid foods from point of spoon or fork, alternated solids and liquids, alternated types of food given to patient, did not blow on food to cool it or taste patient's food, allowed patient to hold bread or assisted if necessary, allowed for rest periods, and used napkin to wipe patient's mouth as needed. ____ ____ _____

30. Removed tray when finished. ____ ____ _____

31. Offered oral hygiene, bedpan, or handwashing as needed. ____ ____ _____

32. Raised side rail if needed. ____ ____ _____

33. Removed gloves and washed hands. ____ ____ _____

34. Documented. ____ ____ _____

**Performance Checklist
Skill 25–2**

ADMINISTERING NASOGASTRIC TUBE AND GASTROSTOMY FEEDINGS

	S	U	Comments
1. Obtained equipment.	___	___	_____
2. Referred to medical record, care plan, or Kardex for special interventions.	___	___	_____
3. Introduced self.	___	___	_____
4. Identified patient by identification band.	___	___	_____
5. Explained procedure to patient.	___	___	_____
6. Washed hands and donned clean gloves.	___	___	_____
7. Prepared patient for intervention.	___	___	_____
8. Raised bed to comfortable working level.	___	___	_____
9. Arranged for patient privacy.	___	___	_____
10. Placed patient in high semi-Fowler's position.	___	___	_____
11. Assessed bowel sounds.	___	___	_____
12. Verified tube placement.	___	___	_____

Intermittent Feeding

	S	U	Comments
13. Filled feeding bag and tubing with formula.	___	___	_____
14. Attached feeding bag to nasogastric tube, regulating drip rate with roller clamp.	___	___	_____
15. Hung feeding bag on intravenous poll 18 inches above patient.	___	___	_____
16. Allowed feeding to infuse slowly for 20 to 30 minutes.	___	___	_____
17. When feeding was completed, flushed nasogastric tube with 30 to 50 ml of water as prescribed.	___	___	_____
18. Clamped nasogastric tube and kept patient comfortable in Fowler's position.	___	___	_____
19. Washed feeding bag and tubing with warm, soapy water; rinsed well; and dried or obtained disposable feeding bag for next feeding.	___	___	_____
20. Gave water between feedings as prescribed.	___	___	_____

	S	U	Comments

Continuous Feeding

21. Filled bag and pump tubing, attached tubing to nasogastric tube, set enteral infusion pump to deliver required volume and rate, unclamped tubing and started pump, and assessed volume every 1 to 2 hours or according to agency policy.

22. Irrigated tube every 3 to 4 hours with 20 to 30 ml of water as prescribed.

Gastrostomy Tube Feeding

23. Placed patient in high semi-Fowler's position.

24. Assessed bowel sounds.

25. Verified tube placement.

26. Determined amount of residual fluid.

27. Returned residual fluid to stomach.

28. Followed procedure for intermittent feeding or continuous feeding and clamped tubing.

29. Cleansed and dressed skin area around gastrostomy tube insertion site as needed.

30. Maintained patient in high semi-Fowler's position.

31. Gave water between feedings as prescribed.

32. Removed gloves and washed hands.

33. Documented.

Performance Checklist
Skill 25–3

ADMINISTERING TOTAL PARENTERAL NUTRITION

	S	U	Comments
1. Obtained equipment.	___	___	_____
2. Referred to medical record, care plan, or Kardex for special interventions.	___	___	_____
3. Introduced self.	___	___	_____
4. Identified patient by identification band.	___	___	_____
5. Explained procedure to patient.	___	___	_____
6. Washed hands and donned clean gloves.	___	___	_____
7. Prepared patient for intervention.	___	___	_____
8. Raised bed to comfortable working level.	___	___	_____
9. Arranged for patient privacy.	___	___	_____
10. Compared total parenteral nutrition label with patient's identification band.	___	___	_____
11. Identified catheter port for total parenteral nutrition, and if necessary, closed it with infusion plug.	___	___	_____
12. Removed cap from filtered intravenous tubing to expose spike.	___	___	_____
13. Removed cover or cap from total parenteral nutrition bottle or bag.	___	___	_____
14. Inserted tubing spike.	___	___	_____
15. Opened drip controller, primed drip chamber, and ran solution through tubing.	___	___	_____
16. Closed drip controller.	___	___	_____
17. Hung feeding bottle or bag on intravenous feeding pole attached to infusion pump.	___	___	_____
18. Slid tubing into infusion pump.	___	___	_____
19. Prepared lipid solution if ordered by inserting vented, nonfiltered tubing spike into lipid bottle; opened drip chamber and ran solution through tubing; and placed 21-gauge needle on end of tubing and plugged into distal port of total parenteral nutrition tubing.	___	___	_____

	S	U	Comments

20. Attached total parenteral nutrition tubing to central catheter port.

    ———— ———— ————————————————

21. Set infusion pump for appropriate volume per hour.

    ———— ———— ————————————————

22. Calculated and assessed drip rate for total parenteral nutrition and lipids if prescribed.

    ———— ———— ————————————————

23. Assisted patient to comfortable position.

    ———— ———— ————————————————

24. Removed used disposable supplies.

    ———— ———— ————————————————

25. Removed gloves and washed hands.

    ———— ———— ————————————————

26. Documented.

    ———— ———— ————————————————

**Performance Checklist
Skill 26–1**

PROMOTING SLEEP

	S	U	Comments
1. Obtained equipment.	___	___	_____
2. Referred to medical record, care plan, or Kardex for special interventions.	___	___	_____
3. Introduced self.	___	___	_____
4. Identified patient by identification band.	___	___	_____
5. Explained procedure to patient.	___	___	_____
6. Washed hands and donned clean gloves.	___	___	_____
7. Prepared patient for intervention.	___	___	_____
8. Raised bed to comfortable working level.	___	___	_____
9. Arranged for patient privacy.	___	___	_____
10. Assessed patient regarding sleep habits, medications currently taking, rituals or routines used at home to aid sleep, and signs and symptoms of sleep deprivation or disturbance.	___	___	_____
11. Explained importance of adequate rest and sleep to patient, especially in relation to healing and restorative functions.	___	___	_____
12. Interviewed patient for revelation of sleep disturbances.	___	___	_____
13. Decided which patient routines that aid in producing sleep at home may be used while in hospital.	___	___	_____
14. Ensured that patient's bedtime was quiet and unhurried and that basic physical and safety needs were met before sleep.	___	___	_____
15. Removed gloves and washed hands.	___	___	_____
16. Documented.	___	___	_____

Performance Checklist
Skill 27–1

RELIEVING PAIN WITH EQUIPMENT AND COMFORT MEASURES

	S	U	Comments
1. Obtained equipment.	___	___	_____
2. Referred to medical record, care plan, or Kardex for special interventions.	___	___	_____
3. Introduced self.	___	___	_____
4. Identified patient by identification band.	___	___	_____
5. Explained procedure to patient.	___	___	_____
6. Washed hands and donned clean gloves.	___	___	_____
7. Prepared patient for intervention.	___	___	_____
8. Raised bed to comfortable working level.	___	___	_____
9. Arranged for patient privacy.	___	___	_____
10. Assessed pain.	___	___	_____

Transcutaneous Electrical Nerve Stimulation (TENS)

	S	U	Comments
11. Positioned electrodes.	___	___	_____
12. Lowered settings before turning unit on.	___	___	_____
13. Increased settings on unit until patient experienced mild to moderate tingling, buzzing, or vibrating sensations.	___	___	_____

Patient-Controlled Analgesia (PCA)

	S	U	Comments
14. Attached PCA to syringe and filled tubing to Y-connector.	___	___	_____
15. Attached intravenous solution tubing to PCA and filled to Y-connector.	___	___	_____
16. Inserted syringe into PCA infuser.	___	___	_____
17. Programmed infuser with beginning dose (bolus), maintenance dose, and lockout interval; programmed intravenous pump as to volume and rate.	___	___	_____
18. Closed security cover and locked with key.	___	___	_____

	S	U	Comments

19. Performed venipuncture if intravenous did not already exist.

    _____ _____ _____

20. Connected PCA to venipuncture device and began intravenous infusion; unclamped PCA tubing.

    _____ _____ _____

Back Massage

21. Positioned patient in prone position.

    _____ _____ _____

22. Draped patient to expose only area to be massaged.

    _____ _____ _____

23. Applied liberal amount of lotion to hands and rubbed palms to warm lotion; reapplied lotion as needed throughout procedure.

    _____ _____ _____

24. Began massage in lower back moving up spine and out over shoulders in circular motion using long, firm strokes for about 3 to 5 minutes.

    _____ _____ _____

25. Massaged buttocks using palm of hand rubbing with circular motion.

    _____ _____ _____

26. Removed any excess lotion from skin.

    _____ _____ _____

27. Repositioned and realigned patient.

    _____ _____ _____

28. Removed gloves and washed hands.

    _____ _____ _____

29. Disposed of waste materials.

    _____ _____ _____

30. Documented.

    _____ _____ _____

Performance Checklist
Skill 28–1

ASSISTING WITH APPLYING SKELETAL TRACTION

	S	U	Comments
1. Obtained equipment.	___	___	_____
2. Referred to medical record, care plan, or Kardex for special interventions.	___	___	_____
3. Introduced self.	___	___	_____
4. Identified patient by identification band.	___	___	_____
5. Explained procedure to patient.	___	___	_____
6. Washed hands and donned clean gloves.	___	___	_____
7. Prepared patient for intervention.	___	___	_____
8. Raised bed to comfortable working level.	___	___	_____
9. Arranged for patient privacy.	___	___	_____
10. Assessed patient for pain; immobility problems; circulation, motion, and sensation to distal extremity; skin condition around pin or tong insertion sites; cleanliness and dryness of dressing; and traction alignment.	___	___	_____
11. Inspected traction apparatus for direction of pull, unobstructed ropes, appropriate alignment of ropes and pulleys, free moving weights, appropriate weight poundage, and secure knots.	___	___	_____
12. Performed color, movement, and sensation (CMS) assessment bilaterally every 2 hours for initial 24 hours and then every 2 to 4 hours.	___	___	_____
13. Maintained extremity in neutral alignment.	___	___	_____
14. Assessed position of Pearson attachment.	___	___	_____
15. Assessed skin around Thomas splint.	___	___	_____
16. Inspected skin or tong sites for localized warmth.	___	___	_____
17. Assessed vital signs every 4 to 8 hours.	___	___	_____
18. Used sterile technique to clean pin sites with hydrogen peroxide or normal saline every shift or according to agency policy.	___	___	_____

	S	U	Comments

19. Cleansed around pin entrance and exit sites with sterile cotton applicators without digging at sites.

_____ _____ _____

20. Applied antibacterial ointment if prescribed.

_____ _____ _____

21. Instructed patient or performed range-of-motion exercises to unaffected muscles and joints every 4 hours.

_____ _____ _____

22. Taught patient strengthening exercises to quadriceps, gluteus triceps, and biceps and had patient perform 10 repetitions every 2 to 4 hours when ordered.

_____ _____ _____

23. Disposed of equipment or waste materials.

_____ _____ _____

24. Removed gloves and washed hands.

_____ _____ _____

25. Documented.

_____ _____ _____

**Performance Checklist
Skill 28–2**

ASSISTING WITH APPLYING SKIN TRACTION

	S	U	Comments
1. Obtained equipment.	___	___	_____
2. Referred to medical record, care plan, or Kardex for special interventions.	___	___	_____
3. Introduced self.	___	___	_____
4. Identified patient by identification band.	___	___	_____
5. Explained procedure to patient.	___	___	_____
6. Washed hands and donned clean gloves.	___	___	_____
7. Prepared patient for intervention.	___	___	_____
8. Raised bed to comfortable working level.	___	___	_____
9. Arranged for patient privacy.	___	___	_____
10. Assessed patient for color, movement, and sensation (CMS) distal to extremity, redness of skin and bony prominences, appropriate body alignment, and high-risk immobility problems.	___	___	_____
11. Placed bed in appropriate position: flat or Trendelenburg.	___	___	_____
12. Cleansed skin with warm, soapy water and rinsed, and dried skin thoroughly.	___	___	_____
13. Assisted physician to apply nonadhesive traction tapes on opposite sides of affected extremity, leaving 4 to 6 inches beyond foot.	___	___	_____
14. Placed padding over bony prominences.	___	___	_____
15. Had second nurse elevate extremity and wrap it in ace bandages.	___	___	_____
16. Assisted with attachment of spreader bar to distal end on nonadhesive traction tapes.	___	___	_____
17. Threaded rope through pulleys and tied correct traction knots.	___	___	_____
18. Tied rope to spreader bar, slowly and gently attached 4 to 7 lbs of weight to distal end of rope.	___	___	_____

	S	**U**	**Comments**

19. Palpated area over adhesive tapes daily. _____ _____ _____

20. While second nurse applied manual traction, removed ace bandages every shift if prescribed. _____ _____ _____

21. Performed CMS assessment bilaterally every 2 to 4 hours. _____ _____ _____

22. Assessed for pressure over peroneal nerve and Achilles tendon every shift. _____ _____ _____

23. Maintained extremity in neutral alignment. _____ _____ _____

24. Assessed for complaints of burning sensation. _____ _____ _____

25. Assessed traction apparatus for direction of pull, unobstructed ropes, free moving weights, and secured knots. _____ _____ _____

26. Assessed patient's comfort and position. _____ _____ _____

27. Placed call light and personal articles within reach. _____ _____ _____

28. Disposed of or cleaned equipment to be returned according to agency policy. _____ _____ _____

29. Removed gloves and washed hands. _____ _____ _____

30. Documented. _____ _____ _____

**Performance Checklist
Skill 28–3**

CARING FOR A CAST

		S	U	Comments
1.	Obtained equipment.	___	___	_____
2.	Referred to medical record, care plan, or Kardex for special interventions.	___	___	_____
3.	Introduced self.	___	___	_____
4.	Identified patient by identification band.	___	___	_____
5.	Explained procedure to patient.	___	___	_____
6.	Washed hands and donned clean gloves.	___	___	_____
7.	Prepared patient for intervention.	___	___	_____
8.	Raised bed to comfortable working level.	___	___	_____
9.	Arranged for patient privacy.	___	___	_____
10.	Assessed patient for newly applied cast, color, movement, and sensation (CMS) distal to extremity, and pain in area where cast was applied.	___	___	_____
11.	Used palms of hands to move extremity or body with newly applied cast.	___	___	_____
12.	Removed bed covers from cast until dried.	___	___	_____
13.	Elevated casted extremity above level of heart on firm pillows, placing them from furrow of buttocks to foot, allowing foot to hang free of pillow, unless contraindicated.	___	___	_____
14.	Performed CMS assessment bilaterally every 1 to 2 hours for initial 24 hours, and then performed assessment every 2 to 4 hours.	___	___	_____
15.	Assessed for signs and symptoms of infection.	___	___	_____
16.	Assessed for blood stains over fracture site and documented date, time, and size of area.	___	___	_____
17.	Inspected for skin irritation around cast edges and petal edges if necessary.	___	___	_____
18.	Assessed for increased pain on passive movement of digits.	___	___	_____

	S	U	Comments

19. Assisted patient to change positions and performed range-of-motion exercises on unaffected extremity. _____ _____ _____

20. Disposed of equipment. _____ _____ _____

21. Removed gloves and washed hands. _____ _____ _____

22. Documented. _____ _____ _____

Performance Checklist
Skill 28–4

APPLYING BRACES

		S	U	Comments
1.	Obtained equipment.	___	___	_____
2.	Referred to medical record, care plan, or Kardex for special interventions.	___	___	_____
3.	Introduced self.	___	___	_____
4.	Identified patient by identification band.	___	___	_____
5.	Explained procedure to patient.	___	___	_____
6.	Washed hands and donned clean gloves.	___	___	_____
7.	Prepared patient for intervention.	___	___	_____
8.	Raised bed to comfortable working level.	___	___	_____
9.	Arranged for patient privacy.	___	___	_____
10.	Assessed patient for skin breakdown, safety of brace device, and need for other assistive devices.	___	___	_____
11.	Had patient wear flat, nonskid shoes.	___	___	_____
12.	Had patient wear thin, knitted undershirt with back brace.	___	___	_____
13.	Had patient lie on bed, fitted brace over appropriate body part, and fastened in place.	___	___	_____
14.	Assisted patient to sitting position on side of bed.	___	___	_____
15.	Assisted patient to ambulate with brace in place.	___	___	_____
16.	Assessed color, movement, and sensation (CMS) to distal extremity every 4 to 8 hours.	___	___	_____
17.	Inspected skin areas after removing brace.	___	___	_____
18.	Placed brace against wall or on table.	___	___	_____
19.	Taught patient to apply and remove brace.	___	___	_____
20.	Disposed of, cleaned, or stored equipment.	___	___	_____
21.	Removed gloves and washed hands.	___	___	_____
22.	Documented.	___	___	_____

Performance Checklist
Skill 28–5

APPLYING AN ABDUCTION PILLOW

	S	U	Comments
1. Obtained equipment.	___	___	_____
2. Referred to medical record, care plan, or Kardex for special interventions.	___	___	_____
3. Introduced self.	___	___	_____
4. Identified patient by identification band.	___	___	_____
5. Explained procedure to patient.	___	___	_____
6. Washed hands and donned clean gloves.	___	___	_____
7. Prepared patient for intervention.	___	___	_____
8. Raised bed to comfortable working level.	___	___	_____
9. Arranged for patient privacy.	___	___	_____
10. Assessed patient for appropriate body posture and neutral alignment of affected leg and hip, redness or open areas of lower extremities, and color, movement, and sensation (CMS) bilaterally of lower extremities.	___	___	_____
11. Placed patient in appropriate posture, with hip and leg in neutral alignment.	___	___	_____
12. Moved patient's nonoperative leg away from legs.	___	___	_____
13. Placed narrow (top) end of abduction pillow near top of patient's thigh but below perineum with velcro straps unfastened.	___	___	_____
14. Placed velcro straps around legs and fastened to top of abduction pillow.	___	___	_____
15. Assessed patient's level of comfort and alignment.	___	___	_____
16. Disposed of waste materials.	___	___	_____
17. Removed gloves and washed hands.	___	___	_____
18. Documented.	___	___	_____

Performance Checklist
Skill 28–6

TEACHING CRUTCH GAITS

	S	U	Comments
1. Obtained equipment.	___	___	_____
2. Referred to medical record, care plan, or Kardex for special interventions.	___	___	_____
3. Introduced self.	___	___	_____
4. Identified patient by identification band.	___	___	_____
5. Explained procedure to patient.	___	___	_____
6. Washed hands and donned clean gloves.	___	___	_____
7. Prepared patient for intervention.	___	___	_____
8. Raised bed to comfortable working level.	___	___	_____
9. Arranged for patient privacy.	___	___	_____
10. Assessed patient for arm and upper body strength, and visual acuity, and crutches for secure attachment of rubber tips, cracks in wood, and abnormal bends in aluminum.	___	___	_____
11. Had patient wear flat, nonskid shoes.	___	___	_____

Standing

12. Instructed patient to place crutches in hand on side, slide forward in straight chair, grasp chair arm with opposite hand, and push up to a standing position.	___	___	_____
13. Had patient assume tripod stance.	___	___	_____
14. Instructed patient in one of four crutch gaits:	___	___	_____

Two-point Gait

15. Had patient move right foot and left crutch forward.	___	___	_____
16. Had patient move left foot and right crutch forward.	___	___	_____

Three-point Gait

17. Had patient stand on stronger leg while moving crutches and weaker leg forward 6 inches.	___	___	_____

	S	**U**	**Comments**

18. Had patient shift weight to crutches and move stronger leg forward.   _____ _____ _____

Swing-through Gait

19. Had patient move crutches forward and then swing legs forward and then swing legs forward in front of crutches.   _____ _____ _____

20. Had patient move crutches forward.   _____ _____ _____

Four-point Gait

21. Had patient move right crutch forward, advance left foot, move left crutch forward, and advance right foot.   _____ _____ _____

Climbing Stairs

22. Had patient place body weight on hand rests of crutches and then move strong leg up to next step.   _____ _____ _____

23. Had patient place weight on crutches and move weaker leg up to next step.   _____ _____ _____

24. Had patient repeat sequence until stairs were ascended.   _____ _____ _____

Descending Stairs

25. Had patient move crutches to lower step; then had patient place weaker leg first, followed by stronger leg.   _____ _____ _____

26. Had patient repeat sequence until stairs were descended.   _____ _____ _____

Sitting

27. Had patient turn around and back toward chair until legs touched chair seat.   _____ _____ _____

28. Had patient place crutches in hand on strong side and, using other hand, grasp chair arm to lower body into chair.   _____ _____ _____

29. Removed gloves and washed hands.   _____ _____ _____

30. Documented.   _____ _____ _____

**Performance Checklist
Skill 28–7**

TEACHING USE OF A CANE

	S	U	Comments
1. Obtained equipment.	___	___	_____
2. Referred to medical record, care plan, or Kardex for special interventions.	___	___	_____
3. Introduced self.	___	___	_____
4. Identified patient by identification band.	___	___	_____
5. Explained procedure to patient.	___	___	_____
6. Washed hands and donned clean gloves.	___	___	_____
7. Prepared patient for intervention.	___	___	_____
8. Raised bed to comfortable working level.	___	___	_____
9. Arranged for patient privacy.	___	___	_____
10. Assessed patient for strength and tightness of patient's handgrip, balance and coordination, strength of unaffected side, visual acuity, and integrity of cane being used.	___	___	_____
11. Measured and adjusted height of cane for aluminum canes.	___	___	_____
12. Had patient wear flat, nonskid shoes.	___	___	_____

Standing and walking

	S	U	Comments
13. Instructed patient to place cane in hand opposite affected leg and slide forward in chair.	___	___	_____
14. Had patient grasp one arm of chair with free hand and, if possible, grasp cane and chair arm with opposite hand or patient can grasp cane only.	___	___	_____
15. Had patient use chair arms and cane to push directly downward to a standing position.	___	___	_____
16. Had patient pause to attain balance before positioning cane once standing.	___	___	_____
17. Had patient stand straight and look ahead.	___	___	_____

	S	**U**	**Comments**

18. Had patient move cane forward 4 to 6 inches and bear weight on unaffected foot while moving cane and affected foot forward simultaneously.   ____ ____ _____

19. Had patient transfer weight to affected foot and cane while moving unaffected foot forward.   ____ ____ _____

20. Walked to side and slightly behind patient.   ____ ____ _____

21. Advised patient to take small steps.   ____ ____ _____

Sitting

22. Had patient use cane to turn around and back into chair until legs touched chair seat.   ____ ____ _____

23. Had patient grasp both chair arms while holding cane in one hand and lowered body into chair.   ____ ____ _____

24. Taught patient to place cane on chair arm.   ____ ____ _____

Climbing stairs

25. Had patient place cane on affected side.   ____ ____ _____

26. Had patient place stronger foot on step while grasping handrail with stronger hand.   ____ ____ _____

27. Had patient shift weight to stronger leg and then move weaker leg onto step.   ____ ____ _____

28. Repeated sequence until stairs were ascended.   ____ ____ _____

Descending stairs

29. Had patient place cane on weaker side and grasp handrail with stronger hand.   ____ ____ _____

30. Had patient move weaker leg and cane to next step.   ____ ____ _____

31. Had patient move strong leg to same step using cane and handrail.   ____ ____ _____

32. Repeated sequence until stairs were descended.   ____ ____ _____

33. Disposed of waste materials.   ____ ____ _____

34. Removed gloves and washed hands.   ____ ____ _____

35. Documented.   ____ ____ _____

**Performance Checklist
Skill 28–8**

TEACHING USE OF A WALKER

		S	U	Comments
1.	Obtained equipment.	___	___	_____
2.	Referred to medical record, care plan, or Kardex for special interventions.	___	___	_____
3.	Introduced self.	___	___	_____
4.	Identified patient by identification band.	___	___	_____
5.	Explained procedure to patient.	___	___	_____
6.	Washed hands and donned clean gloves.	___	___	_____
7.	Prepared patient for intervention.	___	___	_____
8.	Raised bed to comfortable working level.	___	___	_____
9.	Arranged for patient privacy.	___	___	_____
10.	Selected appropriate walker and adjusted walker height if necessary.	___	___	_____
11.	Had patient wear flat, nonskid shoes.	___	___	_____
12.	Placed walker in front of patient.	___	___	_____
13.	Had patient place both hands on chair arms, slide forward, and push up to standing position.	___	___	_____
14.	Had patient place one hand at a time on walker handgrips.	___	___	_____
15.	Had patient shift weight to unaffected leg while walker and affected leg are simultaneously moved forward 4 to 6 inches.	___	___	_____
16.	Had patient shift weight to walker and affected leg and move stronger leg forward.	___	___	_____
17.	Repeated sequence for anticipated distance.	___	___	_____
18.	Walked closely behind and slightly to side of patient.	___	___	_____

Sitting

- Had patient turn around in front of chair and back up until legs touched chair. ___ ___ _____

	S	U	Comments

- Had patient shift weight to stronger leg and reach behind with one hand and then other hand to grasp chair arms. _____ _____ _____

- Had patient bear weight on chair arms and lower into chair. _____ _____ _____

- Placed walker beside chair. _____ _____ _____

19. Removed gloves and washed hands. _____ _____ _____

20. Documented. _____ _____ _____

Performance Checklist
Skill 28–9

USING A WHEELCHAIR

		S	U	Comments
1.	Obtained equipment.	___	___	_____
2.	Referred to medical record, care plan, or Kardex for special interventions.	___	___	_____
3.	Introduced self.	___	___	_____
4.	Identified patient by identification band.	___	___	_____
5.	Explained procedure to patient.	___	___	_____
6.	Washed hands and donned clean gloves.	___	___	_____
7.	Prepared patient for intervention.	___	___	_____
8.	Raised bed to comfortable working level.	___	___	_____
9.	Arranged for patient privacy.	___	___	_____
10.	Assessed patient for arm and shoulder strength, leg strength, redness of skin and bony prominences, and motivation to regain independence.	___	___	_____

Transfer by lifting

		S	U	Comments
11.	Positioned wheelchair beside bed, locked brakes, and lifted up footrests.	___	___	_____
12.	Removed armrests, raised patient's head, and raised bed above level of chair.	___	___	_____
13.	Crossed patient's hands over chest and arranged nurses for procedure.	___	___	_____
14.	Counted to 3 and nurses simultaneously lifted patient into wheelchair.	___	___	_____
15.	Placed patient in appropriate body alignment.	___	___	_____
16.	Applied restraining device or lap belt on patients with altered level of consciousness or quadriplegia.	___	___	_____

Transfer by pivoting

		S	U	Comments
17.	Positioned wheelchair beside bed on patient's stronger side, locked brakes, and lifted up footrests.	___	___	_____

	S	U	Comments

18. Assisted patient to sitting position on side of bed.

19. Placed arms under axillae and grasped hands behind patient's back while moving in front of patient.

20. Had patient use strong leg to assist in standing.

21. Allowed patient few seconds to gain balance.

22. Nurse and patient pivoted together; backed patient up to chair; had patient grasp chair arms and lowered into wheelchair.

23. Unlocked brakes and pushed wheelchair in direction patient is facing.

24. Pushed wheelchair in normal manner if descending a gently sloped ramp.

25. Turned wheelchair around and descended backward if descending a steep ramp.

26. Removed gloves and washed hands.

27. Documented.

**Performance Checklist
Skill 28–10**

USING A THERAPEUTIC FRAME OR BED

	S	U	Comments
1. Obtained equipment.	___	___	_____
2. Referred to medical record, care plan, or Kardex for special interventions.	___	___	_____
3. Introduced self.	___	___	_____
4. Identified patient by identification band.	___	___	_____
5. Explained procedure to patient.	___	___	_____
6. Washed hands and donned clean gloves.	___	___	_____
7. Prepared patient for intervention.	___	___	_____
8. Raised bed to comfortable working level.	___	___	_____
9. Arranged for patient privacy.	___	___	_____
10. Assessed patient for level of anxiety and apprehension, level of pain, need for elimination, vital signs and respiratory status, intake within last 15 to 20 minutes, and safety of bed being used.	___	___	_____

Frame

	S	U	Comments
11. Removed all accessories, including bedpan, and secured intravenous bags and lines, urinary catheter bags, or other drainage bags.	___	___	_____
12. Placed pillows across patient's chest and any areas where sliding is possible.	___	___	_____
13. With two people, placed anterior or posterior frame over patient and fastened ends of frame together with screws.	___	___	_____
14. Placed two safety straps around anterior and posterior frames and patient, one over chest and other over thighs.	___	___	_____
15. Double-checked all screws, bolts, and straps.	___	___	_____
16. Informed patient of direction of turn.	___	___	_____
17. Arranged a signal so that patient would know when frame would be turned.	___	___	_____

	S	U	Comments

18. On count of 3, turned patient in smooth, uninterrupted motion at moderate speed.   ____ ____ _____

19. Removed safety straps and uppermost frame.   ____ ____ _____

20. Assessed patient's position and alignment.   ____ ____ _____

21. Repositioned accessories and placed personal articles and call light within easy reach.   ____ ____ _____

22. Stored frame securely.   ____ ____ _____

23. Repeated turning at least every 2 hours unless physician ordered different schedule.   ____ ____ _____

CircOlectric bed

24. Removed footboard and armrests and secured traction, intravenous bags and lines, urinary catheter bags, other drainage bags, and electric cord.   ____ ____ _____

25. Removed nuts and bolts from both ends of frame.   ____ ____ _____

26. With another nurse, lifted frame over patient, replaced bolts, and tightly secured frame with nuts.   ____ ____ _____

27. Adjusted headrest and padded footboard on uppermost frame if patient was supine.   ____ ____ _____

28. Instructed patient to grasp sides of frame or cross arms over chest.   ____ ____ _____

29. Double-checked nuts and bolts' direction.   ____ ____ _____

30. Informed patient of turning direction.   ____ ____ _____

31. Turned bed without stopping until it reached desired position, using control switch.   ____ ____ _____

32. Second nurse assessed closely for signs of cardiac and respiratory arrest and intravenous line and tube entanglement.   ____ ____ _____

33. Released uppermost frame and applied two safety straps if patient was prone; otherwise, removed uppermost frame.   ____ ____ _____

34. Assessed patient's position, alignment, and face support, and removed wrinkles from sheets.   ____ ____ _____

35. Assessed patient's vital signs.   ____ ____ _____

36. Repositioned accessories and placed personal articles and call light within easy reach.   ____ ____ _____

37. Stored frame securely.   ____ ____ _____

38. Repeated procedure every 2 hours unless contraindicated.   ____ ____ _____

Performance Checklist
Skill 28–10

USING A THERAPEUTIC FRAME OR BED
(Continued)

	S	U	Comments

Roto rest bed

39. Made sure bed was turned off before positioning in bed and locked bed and wheels and latched all hatches.

40. Moved patient to center of bed, smoothed pillow case under hips, placed tubes through designated areas in hatches, and ensured traction was free hanging.

41. Inserted thoracic side supports and allowed 1-inch space between axilla and supports.

42. Pushed supports against chest and locked cam arms securely.

43. Placed disposable supports under patient's legs.

44. Installed and adjusted foot supports to maintain correct position and kept in place only 2 hours every shift.

45. Placed abductor packs in appropriate supports, allowing 6-inch space between packs and patient's groin.

46. Tightened associated knobs.

47. Applied leg supports against hips, positioned knee assemblies slightly above knees, tightened cam arms for leg and knee assemblies, and positioned knee packs until they rested slightly on top of nurse's hand covering patient's knees.

48. Loosened retaining rings on cross bar and carefully slid head and shoulder assembly in place, just touching patient's head; moved shoulder packs until they touched nurse's hand on patient's shoulders, and tightened in place.

	S	U	Comments

49. Tightened head and shoulder assembly tightly so that it would not move off bed, and tightened restraining rings next to shoulder-assembly bracket.

    ____   ____   _____

50. Placed patient's arms on disposable supports, applied side arm supports, and secured safety straps across shoulder assembly and thoracic supports.

    ____   ____   _____

51. Balanced bed as directed in manufacturing instructions.

    ____   ____   _____

52. Assessed that all packs were securely in place.

    ____   ____   _____

53. Held footboard firmly and removed locking pin to start motor.

    ____   ____   _____

54. Raised connecting arm cam handle until connecting assembly locked in place.

    ____   ____   _____

55. Remained with patient for 3 complete turns side to side.

    ____   ____   _____

56. Referred to manufacturer's instructions for placement of drainage tubes through hatches.

    ____   ____   _____

57. Performed scheduled range-of-motion exercises as prescribed.

    ____   ____   _____

58. Locked bed in extreme lateral position for access to back of head, thorax, and buttocks through appropriate hatches.

    ____   ____   _____

Clinitron bed

59. Transferred patient to bed using appropriate transfer techniques.

    ____   ____   _____

60. Assessed patient's position and alignment.

    ____   ____   _____

61. Turned on control for activating fluidization.

    ____   ____   _____

62. Adjusted temperature control.

    ____   ____   _____

63. Replaced covers and placed personal items and call light within easy reach.

    ____   ____   _____

64. Assessed for nausea.

    ____   ____   _____

65. Removed gloves and washed hands.

    ____   ____   _____

66. Documented.

    ____   ____   _____

Performance Checklist
Skill 29–1

USING INCENTIVE SPIROMETRY

	S	U	Comments
1. Obtained equipment.			
2. Referred to medical record, care plan, or Kardex for special interventions.			
3. Introduced self.			
4. Identified patient by identification band.			
5. Explained procedure to patient.			
6. Washed hands and donned clean gloves.			
7. Prepared patient for intervention.			
8. Raised bed to comfortable working level.			
9. Arranged for patient privacy.			
10. Assessed respiratory status.			
11. Placed patient in semi-Fowler's position unless contraindicated.			
12. Taught steps for using spirometer.			
13. Requested patient to insert mouthpiece and inhale slowly and deeply.			
14. Had patient repeat steps required number of times according to medical orders or agency policy.			
15. Offered mouth care.			
16. Cleaned and stored spirometer.			
17. Disposed of waste materials.			
18. Removed gloves and washed hands.			
19. Documented.			

Performance Checklist
Skill 29–2

PERFORMING POSTURAL DRAINAGE AND PERCUSSION

	S	U	Comments
1. Obtained equipment.	___	___	_____
2. Referred to medical record, care plan, or Kardex for special interventions.	___	___	_____
3. Introduced self.	___	___	_____
4. Identified patient by identification band.	___	___	_____
5. Explained procedure to patient.	___	___	_____
6. Washed hands and donned clean gloves.	___	___	_____
7. Prepared patient for intervention.	___	___	_____
8. Raised bed to comfortable working level.	___	___	_____
9. Arranged for patient privacy.	___	___	_____
10. Assessed respiratory status, including breath sounds.	___	___	_____
11. Positioned patient in ordered positions.	___	___	_____
12. Percussed chest wall and back with cupped hand or percussion device.	___	___	_____
13. Vibrated chest wall by placing one hand over the other while patient slowly exhaled.	___	___	_____
14. Provided rest period.	___	___	_____
15. Repeated procedure as prescribed.	___	___	_____
16. Disposed of waste materials.	___	___	_____
17. Removed gloves and washed hands.	___	___	_____
18. Documented.	___	___	_____

Performance Checklist
Skill 29–3

USING THE VAPORIZER

		S	U	Comments
1.	Obtained equipment.	___	___	_____
2.	Referred to medical record, care plan, or Kardex for special interventions.	___	___	_____
3.	Introduced self.	___	___	_____
4.	Identified patient by identification band.	___	___	_____
5.	Explained procedure to patient.	___	___	_____
6.	Washed hands and donned clean gloves.	___	___	_____
7.	Prepared patient for intervention.	___	___	_____
8.	Raised bed to comfortable working level.	___	___	_____
9.	Arranged for patient privacy.	___	___	_____
10.	Assessed respiratory status, including breath sounds.	___	___	_____
11.	Filled vaporizer with distilled water up to indicated line.	___	___	_____
12.	Directed flow of mist toward patient but not directly on patient.	___	___	_____
13.	Adjusted flow and temperature.	___	___	_____
14.	Monitored patient and changed moist clothing as necessary.	___	___	_____
15.	Removed gloves and washed hands.	___	___	_____
16.	Documented.	___	___	_____

**Performance Checklist
Skill 29–4**

ADMINISTERING OXYGEN

	S	U	Comments
1. Obtained equipment.	___	___	_____
2. Referred to medical record, care plan, or Kardex for special interventions.	___	___	_____
3. Introduced self.	___	___	_____
4. Identified patient by identification band.	___	___	_____
5. Explained procedure to patient.	___	___	_____
6. Washed hands and donned clean gloves.	___	___	_____
7. Prepared patient for intervention.	___	___	_____
8. Raised bed to comfortable working level.	___	___	_____
9. Arranged for patient privacy.	___	___	_____
10. Assessed respiratory status, including breath sounds.	___	___	_____
11. Assessed laboratory reports of arterial blood gases.	___	___	_____
12. Applied appropriate type of oxygen.	___	___	_____
13. Provided oral care frequently as needed.	___	___	_____
14. Removed gloves and washed hands.	___	___	_____
15. Documented.	___	___	_____

PERFORMING OROPHARYNGEAL SUCTIONING

	S	U	Comments
1. Obtained equipment.	___	___	_____
2. Referred to medical record, care plan, or Kardex for special interventions.	___	___	_____
3. Introduced self.	___	___	_____
4. Identified patient by identification band.	___	___	_____
5. Explained procedure to patient.	___	___	_____
6. Washed hands and donned clean gloves.	___	___	_____
7. Prepared patient for intervention.	___	___	_____
8. Raised bed to comfortable working level.	___	___	_____
9. Arranged for patient privacy.	___	___	_____
10. Assessed respiratory status, including breath sounds.	___	___	_____
11. Assessed for indications of airway obstruction.	___	___	_____
12. Selected appropriate suction pressure.	___	___	_____
13. Poured sterile solutions into sterile containers.	___	___	_____
14. Attached suction catheter to suction apparatus, touching only thumb-control end and leaving suction tip in package, and turned suction machine on.	___	___	_____
15. Measured approximate length of catheter to insert by noting distance from patient's mouth to earlobe and earlobe to Adam's apple.	___	___	_____
16. Removed one clean glove and replaced with sterile glove.	___	___	_____
17. Held suction tip in sterile gloved hand and thumb-control end in clean hand.	___	U	_____
18. Lubricated suction end by inserting into sterile solution or water-soluble lubricant.	___	___	_____
19. Inserted suction catheter gently into one side of mouth.	___	___	_____

	S	U	Comments

20. Glided catheter toward oropharynx. _____ _____ _____

21. Stopped procedure if met with resistance. _____ _____ _____

22. Placed thumb of clean hand over thumb-control tip, rotating slightly and twisting catheter gently back and forth, as it was withdrawn. _____ _____ _____

23. Limited suction time to 10 to 15 seconds by releasing thumb control. _____ _____ _____

24. Allowed patient to rest and repeated suctioning if necessary. _____ _____ _____

25. Rinsed suction catheter between suctionings by running sterile saline or sterile water through tubing. _____ _____ _____

26. Allowed patient to cough deeply. _____ _____ _____

27. Suctioned between gum line and under tongue. _____ _____ _____

28. Discarded contaminated suction catheter. _____ _____ _____

29. Removed gloves and washed hands. _____ _____ _____

30. Replaced sterile suction catheter for next use. _____ _____ _____

31. Documented. _____ _____ _____

**Performance Checklist
Skill 29–6**

PERFORMING NASOPHARYNGEAL SUCTIONING

	S	U	Comments
1. Obtained equipment.	___	___	_____
2. Referred to medical record, care plan, or Kardex for special interventions.	___	___	_____
3. Introduced self.	___	___	_____
4. Identified patient by identification band.	___	___	_____
5. Explained procedure to patient.	___	___	_____
6. Washed hands and donned clean gloves.	___	___	_____
7. Prepared patient for intervention.	___	___	_____
8. Raised bed to comfortable working level.	___	___	_____
9. Arranged for patient privacy.	___	___	_____
10. Assessed respiratory status, including breath sounds.	___	___	_____
11. Assessed for indications of obstruction.	___	___	_____
12. Selected appropriate suction pressure.	___	___	_____
13. Poured sterile solutions into sterile containers.	___	___	_____
14. Attached suction apparatus to thumb-control end of suction catheter without touching suction end of catheter.	___	___	_____
15. Measured approximate length of catheter by noting distance from nares to earlobe and lobe to Adam's apple.	___	___	_____
16. Left suction end of catheter in sterile package; turned on suction machine.	___	___	_____
17. Removed clean glove and donned sterile glove on dominant hand.	___	___	_____
18. Handled suction end of catheter with sterile hand; handled thumb-control end with clean hand.	___	___	_____
19. Lubricated suction catheter by inserting end into sterile solution.	___	___	_____

	S	U	Comments

20. Inserted suction catheter gently through nose into nasopharynx and stopped procedure if met with resistance at a lower point.

    _____ _____ _____

21. Placed thumb over thumb-control, rotating slightly and twisting catheter back and forth as it was withdrawn.

    _____ _____ _____

22. Limited suction time to 10 to 15 seconds.

    _____ _____ _____

23. Removed thumb from thumb control every 2 to 3 seconds; never suctioned during insertion of catheter.

    _____ _____ _____

24. Allowed patient to rest and repeated suctioning as necessary.

    _____ _____ _____

25. Allowed patient to cough deeply.

    _____ _____ _____

26. Suctioned between gum line and under tongue.

    _____ _____ _____

27. Rinsed catheter by suctioning sterile solution through tubing after each suctioning.

    _____ _____ _____

28. Discarded contaminated suction catheter.

    _____ _____ _____

29. Arranged sterile suction catheter for next use.

    _____ _____ _____

30. Provided oral care as needed.

    _____ _____ _____

31. Removed gloves and washed hands.

    _____ _____ _____

32. Documented.

    _____ _____ _____

Performance Checklist
Skill 29–7

PERFORMING ENDOTRACHEAL SUCTIONING

		S	U	Comments
1.	Obtained equipment.			
2.	Referred to medical record, care plan, or Kardex for special interventions.			
3.	Introduced self.			
4.	Identified patient by identification band.			
5.	Explained procedure to patient.			
6.	Washed hands and donned clean gloves.			
7.	Prepared patient for intervention.			
8.	Raised bed to comfortable working level.			
9.	Arranged for patient privacy.			
10.	Assessed respiratory status, including breath sounds.			
11.	Assessed for indications of airway obstruction.			
12.	Selected appropriate suction pressure.			
13.	Poured sterile solutions into sterile containers.			
14.	Attached suction apparatus to thumb-control end of suction catheter without touching suction end, and left suction end of catheter in sterile package.			
15.	Turned on suction machine.			
16.	Measured approximate length of catheter needed by noting distance from patient's nares to earlobe and lobe to midsternum.			
17.	Removed one clean glove and replaced with sterile glove.			
18.	Held thumb-control end with clean end and suction end of catheter with dominant sterile-gloved hand.			
19.	Lubricated catheter by inserting suction end into sterile solution.			

	S	U	Comments

20. Inserted suction catheter gently through nose into trachea and stopped procedure if met with resistance.

21. Placed thumb over thumb control, rotating slightly and twisting catheter gently back and forth as it was withdrawn.

22. Limited suction time to 10 to 15 seconds and lifted thumb from control every 2 to 3 seconds; did not suction during insertion.

23. Allowed patient to rest and repeated suctioning if necessary.

24. Allowed patient to cough deeply.

25. Suctioned between gum line and under tongue.

26. Rinsed catheter by suctioning sterile solution; performed this after each suctioning.

27. Discarded contaminated suction catheter.

28. Disposed of waste materials.

29. Arranged sterile section catheter for next use.

30. Provided oral care.

31. Removed gloves and washed hands.

32. Documented.

**Performance Checklist
Skill 29–8**

PERFORMING TRACHEOSTOMY CARE AND SUCTIONING

		S	U	Comments
1.	Obtained equipment.	___	___	_____
2.	Referred to medical record, care plan, or Kardex for special interventions.	___	___	_____
3.	Introduced self.	___	___	_____
4.	Identified patient by identification band.	___	___	_____
5.	Explained procedure to patient.	___	___	_____
6.	Washed hands and donned clean gloves.	___	___	_____
7.	Prepared patient for intervention.	___	___	_____
8.	Raised bed to comfortable working level.	___	___	_____
9.	Arranged for patient privacy.	___	___	_____
10.	Assessed respiratory status, including breath sounds.	___	___	_____
11.	Assessed stoma for redness, edema, character of secretions, and bleeding.	___	___	_____
12.	Prepared supplies for suction.	___	___	_____
13.	Placed sterile hemostat, sterile obturator, and sterile tracheostomy set at bedside.	___	___	_____
14.	Attached suction apparatus to thumb-control end of catheter without touching suction end; left suction end in sterile package.	___	___	_____
15.	Poured sterile solutions into sterile containers: hydrogen peroxide into one basin of the tracheostomy cleaning kit and sterile water or saline into the other.	___	___	_____
16.	Placed sterile drape on patient's chest under tracheostomy without touching upper surface of drape.	___	___	_____
17.	Turned on suction machine and adjusted to appropriate level for age.	___	___	_____

	S	**U**	**Comments**

18. Unlocked and removed cannula and placed in basin with hydrogen peroxide.

_____ _____ _____

19. Removed one clean glove and replaced with sterile glove.

_____ _____ _____

20. Held thumb-control end with clean hand and suction end with sterile hand.

_____ _____ _____

21. Lubricated catheter by placing suction end in sterile solution.

_____ _____ _____

22. Instilled small amount of sterile solution into tracheostomy if by medical order.

_____ _____ _____

23. Inserted suction catheter into tracheostomy slowly and gently with no suction applied; stopped if felt resistance.

_____ _____ _____

24. Held thumb over thumb control and pulled catheter out of tracheostomy tube, turning slightly and twisting catheter gently back and forth.

_____ _____ _____

25. Limited suctioning to 10 to 15 seconds and removed thumb from control every 2 to 3 seconds.

_____ _____ _____

26. Allowed patient to rest and repeated suctioning if needed.

_____ _____ _____

27. Administered oxygen between suctionings if needed.

_____ _____ _____

28. Allowed patient to cough deeply.

_____ _____ _____

29. Suctioned around outside edge of tracheostomy tube.

_____ _____ _____

30. Rinsed catheter by suctioning sterile solution; did this after each suctioning.

_____ _____ _____

31. Discarded contaminated catheter.

_____ _____ _____

32. Removed clean gloves and replaced with sterile gloves.

_____ _____ _____

33. Arranged pipe cleaners, brush, gauze pads, forceps, and cotton tapes on sterile field.

_____ _____ _____

34. Picked up inner cannula from peroxide with forceps; used brush and pipe cleaners to thoroughly cleanse inside and outside of cannula; twisted pipe cleaners together or bent double to provide appropriate thickness to fit inside cannula.

_____ _____ _____

35. Rinsed cannula in sterile water.

_____ _____ _____

36. Dried cannula with gauze pads.

_____ _____ _____

**Performance Checklist
Skill 29–8**

PERFORMING TRACHEOSTOMY CARE AND SUCTIONING (Continued)

	S	U	Comments
37. Inspected to ensure cannula was clean and dry inside.	___	___	_____
38. Replaced and locked cannula.	___	___	_____
39. Cleansed skin and surrounding area of stoma with gauze pads moistened with peroxide.	___	___	_____
40. Changed tracheostomy tie tapes if soiled; inserted new tapes before removing old tapes; if this was not possible, had a helper hold tracheostomy tube in place with clean gloved hand while replaced ties.	___	___	_____
41. Replaced soiled gauze pad under tracheostomy tube without dislodging tube.	___	___	_____
42. Provided oral hygiene.	___	___	_____
43. Disposed of all waste materials.	___	___	_____
44. Removed gloves and washed hands.	___	___	_____
45. Documented.	___	___	_____

Performance Checklist
Skill 29–9

CARING FOR CLOSED CHEST DRAINAGE SYSTEMS

	S	U	Comments
1. Obtained equipment.	___	___	_____
2. Referred to medical record, care plan, or Kardex for special interventions.	___	___	_____
3. Introduced self.	___	___	_____
4. Identified patient by identification band.	___	___	_____
5. Explained procedure to patient.	___	___	_____
6. Washed hands and donned clean gloves.	___	___	_____
7. Prepared patient for intervention.	___	___	_____
8. Raised bed to comfortable working level.	___	___	_____
9. Arranged for patient privacy.	___	___	_____
10. Assessed respiratory status, including breath sounds.	___	___	_____
11. Assessed insertion site of chest catheter for leakage, subcutaneous emphysema, and signs of infection.	___	___	_____
12. Assessed all equipment for appropriate working order.	___	___	_____
13. Assessed water level in bottles or disposable setup.	___	___	_____
14. Marked level of drainage, giving date and time.	___	___	_____
15. Made certain tubing does not loop, is not kinked, and does not prevent patient movement.	___	___	_____
16. Encouraged patient movement as allowed and deep breathing and coughing exercises as prescribed; splinted chest to decrease pain.	___	___	_____
17. Kept drainage bottle below chest.	___	___	_____
18. Stripped chest catheter according to agency policy or medical orders.	___	___	_____

	S	U	Comments

19. Made certain there was fluctuation of fluid level in water chamber. ____ ____ _____

20. Made certain there was not a continuous stream of air bubbles in water chamber. ____ ____ _____

21. Reported any of following immediately: shallow breathing, cyanosis, pressure in chest, and hemorrhage. ____ ____ _____

22. If chest tube became disconnected, registered or licensed practical or vocational nurse should use sterile connector to reconnect drainage system. ____ ____ _____

23. If chest tube became dislodged from chest wall, applied pressure with gloved hand and sterile gauze and called for help. ____ ____ _____

24. Disposed of waste materials. ____ ____ _____

25. Removed gloves and washed hands. ____ ____ _____

26. Documented. ____ ____ _____

PERFORMING MALE AND FEMALE CATHETERIZATION

	S	U	Comments

1. Obtained equipment.

2. Referred to medical record, care plan, or Kardex for special interventions.

3. Introduced self.

4. Identified patient by identification band.

5. Explained procedure to patient.

6. Washed hands and donned clean gloves.

7. Prepared patient for intervention.

8. Raised bed to comfortable working level.

9. Arranged for patient privacy.

10. Assisted patient to position.

11. Arranged light.

12. Washed, rinsed, and dried perineum of female if necessary.

13. Removed gloves and washed hands.

14. Placed supplies at foot of bed and opened.

15. Opened sterile gloves.

16. Donned sterile gloves.

17. Placed sterile drape under patient's buttocks and placed cleansing tray near perineum.

18. Opened cleansing agent and poured on all but one or two cotton balls.

19. Removed cap from syringe containing sterile water.

20. Squirted water-soluble lubricant on side near perineum.

21. Placed tray with Foley catheter touching cleansing tray.

	S	U	Comments

Male catheterization

22. Placed sterile fenestrated drape over penis and over upper thighs.

23. Grasped penis in nondominant hand at shaft below glans with one hand holding it up; continued to hold throughout procedure.

24. With dominant hand, used forceps to cleanse penis with cotton balls.

25. Cleansed meatus in circular motions without touching meatus with same cotton ball more than once.

26. Repeated cleansing twice more, using sterile cotton balls each time.

Female catheterization

27. Spread labia minora with thumb and index finger of nondominant hand to expose urinary meatus.

28. With dominant hand, used forceps to hold soaked cotton balls.

29. Cleansed area from clitoris down past anus; next cleansed down right side of labia and then down left side of labia, and cleansed down center once more if necessary.

30. Picked up catheter near tip with dominant hand; kept distal end of catheter in container with closed drainage system.

31. Lubricated tip of catheter and gently inserted 2 to 4 inches (female) and 7 to 9 inches (male) until urine began to flow; then inserted catheter another inch.

32. Collected urine specimen if needed by placing open end of catheter into specimen container.

33. Proceeded according to type catheter:

34. Foley catheter:

   • Inflated balloon with required amount of sterile water.

   • Pulled catheter gently to ensure feeling of resistance.

   • Attached closed drainage system to appropriate place on bed below level of bladder.

   • Secured catheter to patient's thigh (female) or abdomen (male) or according to agency policy.

PERFORMING MALE AND FEMALE CATHETERIZATION (Continued)

	S	U	Comments
• Clipped drainage tubing to bed linen; allowed slack for body movement.	____	____	_____
35. Straight catheter:			
• Held coiled catheter in hand with opening over basin.	____	____	_____
• Emptied bladder completely and removed catheter.	____	____	_____
36. Dried perineal area.	____	____	_____
37. Disposed of supplies.	____	____	_____
38. Labeled urine specimen and took to laboratory with requisition.	____	____	_____
39. Repositioned patient.	____	____	_____
40. Assessed urine flow in drainage bag; noted characteristics of urine.	____	____	_____
41. Removed gloves and washed hands.	____	____	_____
42. Documented.	____	____	_____

Performance Checklist
Skill 30–2

PERFORMING BLADDER IRRIGATION AND INSTILLATION

	S	U	Comments
1. Obtained equipment.	___	___	_____
2. Referred to medical record, care plan, or Kardex for special interventions.	___	___	_____
3. Introduced self.	___	___	_____
4. Identified patient by identification band.	___	___	_____
5. Explained procedure to patient.	___	___	_____
6. Washed hands and donned clean gloves.	___	___	_____
7. Prepared patient for intervention.	___	___	_____
8. Raised bed to comfortable working level.	___	___	_____
9. Arranged for patient privacy.	___	___	_____
10. Placed waterproof pad under patient.	___	___	_____
11. Positioned patient to supine.	___	___	_____
12. Opened sterile supplies and arranged on bedside table.	___	___	_____
13. Poured sterile solution into sterile graduate and recapped solution bottle.	___	___	_____
14. Removed gloves, washed hands, and donned sterile gloves.	___	___	_____
15. Placed sterile basin between patient's legs, near perineal area.	___	___	_____
16. Disconnected catheter from drainage system and plugged end of catheter or used port of closed drainage system.	___	___	_____
17. Cleansed end of catheter with antiseptic swab.	___	___	_____

Irrigation

	S	U	Comments
18. Drew 30-ml sterile solution into syringe.	___	___	_____
19. Placed tip of syringe into end of catheter and injected solution slowly.	___	___	_____

	S	U	Comments

20. Withdrew syringe, allowing solution to drain by gravity into basin.

_____ _____ _____

21. Repeated until either all solution had been used or solution was clear.

_____ _____ _____

22. Reattached drainage system if needed.

_____ _____ _____

23. Assessed and measured drainage.

_____ _____ _____

24. Disposed of waste materials.

_____ _____ _____

Instillation

25. Drew medication or solution into syringe.

_____ _____ _____

26. Placed tip of syringe into end of catheter and slowly injected solution.

_____ _____ _____

27. Clamped off end of catheter for period of time necessary.

_____ _____ _____

28. Removed gloves and washed hands.

_____ _____ _____

29. Documented.

_____ _____ _____

Performance Checklist
Skill 30–3

COLLECTING A STERILE URINE SPECIMEN
FROM A FOLEY CATHETER

		S	U	Comments
1.	Obtained equipment.	___	___	_____
2.	Referred to medical record, care plan, or Kardex for special interventions.	___	___	_____
3.	Introduced self.	___	___	_____
4.	Identified patient by identification band.	___	___	_____
5.	Explained procedure to patient.	___	___	_____
6.	Washed hands and donned clean gloves.	___	___	_____
7.	Prepared patient for intervention.	___	___	_____
8.	Raised bed to comfortable working level.	___	___	_____
9.	Arranged for patient privacy.	___	___	_____
10.	Clamped tubing to allow urine to collect.	___	___	_____
11.	Cleansed catheter port with antiseptic swab.	___	___	_____
12.	Inserted needle into port at 30- to 45-degree angle, watching for needle tip to enter tubing lumen.	___	___	_____
13.	Aspirated 5- to 10-ml urine into syringe and removed needle.	___	___	_____
14.	Placed urine in sterile container.	___	___	_____
15.	Disposed of used syringe into required container.	___	___	_____
16.	Rewiped port with swab.	___	___	_____
17.	Unclamped catheter tubing.	___	___	_____
18.	Labeled specimen appropriately.	___	___	_____
19.	Removed gloves and washed hands.	___	___	_____
20.	Documented.	___	___	_____

Performance Checklist
Skill 31–1

REMOVING A FECAL IMPACTION

		S	U	Comments
1.	Obtained equipment.	____	____	
2.	Referred to medical record, care plan, or Kardex for special interventions.	____	____	
3.	Introduced self.	____	____	
4.	Identified patient by identification band.	____	____	
5.	Explained procedure to patient.	____	____	
6.	Washed hands and donned clean gloves.	____	____	
7.	Prepared patient for intervention.	____	____	
8.	Raised bed to comfortable working height.	____	____	
9.	Arranged for patient privacy.	____	____	
10.	Placed patient in left Sims' position.	____	____	
11.	Placed waterproof pad under patient's buttocks.	____	____	
12.	Placed bedpan on bed near foot of bed.	____	____	
13.	Arranged patient's gown and top linen out of way yet providing privacy.	____	____	
14.	Counted radial pulse.	____	____	
15.	Lubricated dominant forefinger liberally.	____	____	
16.	Inserted forefinger gently into rectum; slowly moved finger into and around fecal mass.	____	____	
17.	As pieces of stool were broken off, removed them to bedpan.	____	____	
18.	Continued procedure until as much as possible of impaction was removed.	____	____	
19.	During procedure, stopped a few minutes if patient complained of discomfort.	____	____	
20.	Following procedure, washed and dried perineal area thoroughly.	____	____	

	S	U	Comments
21. Removed waterproof pad and repositioned patient to comfort.	___	___	_____
22. Disposed of equipment.	___	___	_____
23. Removed gloves and washed hands.	___	___	_____
24. Counted radial pulse.	___	___	_____
25. Documented.	___	___	_____

Performance Checklist
Skill 31–2

PERFORMING BOWEL TRAINING

	S	U	Comments
1. Obtained equipment.	___	___	_____
2. Referred to medical record, care plan, or Kardex for special interventions.	___	___	_____
3. Introduced self.	___	___	_____
4. Identified patient by identification band.	___	___	_____
5. Explained procedure to patient.	___	___	_____
6. Washed hands and donned clean gloves.	___	___	_____
7. Prepared patient for intervention.	___	___	_____
8. Raised bed to comfortable working level.	___	___	_____
9. Arranged for patient privacy.	___	___	_____
10. Asked patient what measures had promoted bowel elimination in past.	___	___	_____
11. Assessed patient's ability to understand and cooperate with program.	___	___	_____
12. Administered cathartic rectal suppository if prescribed 30 minutes before normal time for defecation.	___	___	_____
13. Provided for factors that normally precede patient's bowel elimination.	___	___	_____
14. Within 30 minutes of suppository administration or earlier if patient expressed urge to defecate, assisted patient to bedpan, bedside commode, or preferably, commode.	___	___	_____
15. Ensured patient privacy and safety by leaving alone no longer than 15 to 30 minutes if condition warranted.	___	___	_____
16. Provided encouragement and positive reinforcement for patient success.	___	___	_____

	S	U	Comments
17. Assisted in cleansing and helping patient back to bed.	___	___	_____
18. Disposed of equipment.	___	___	_____
19. Removed gloves and washed hands.	___	___	_____
20. Documented.	___	___	_____

**Performance Checklist
Skill 31–3**

INSERTING A RECTAL TUBE

	S	U	Comments
1. Obtained equipment.	___	___	_____
2. Referred to medical record, care plan, or Kardex for special interventions.	___	___	_____
3. Introduced self.	___	___	_____
4. Identified patient by identification band.	___	___	_____
5. Explained procedure to patient.	___	___	_____
6. Washed hands and donned clean gloves.	___	___	_____
7. Prepared patient for intervention.	___	___	_____
8. Raised bed to comfortable working level.	___	___	_____
9. Arranged for patient privacy.	___	___	_____
10. Had patient assume left side-lying position.	___	___	_____
11. Arranged gown and top linens out of way yet draping patient.	___	___	_____
12. Placed waterproof pad under patient's buttocks.	___	___	_____
13. Lubricated rectal tube thoroughly.	___	___	_____
14. Exposed anus to view and inserted rectal tube 4 to 6 inches (10 to 15 cm), avoiding injury.	___	___	_____
15. Taped tube to buttocks and inserted end into receptacle or used commercially prepared setup.	___	___	_____
16. Instructed patient to lie still.	___	___	_____
17. Left rectal tube in place no longer than 30 minutes at one time.	___	___	_____
18. Removed rectal tube and assisted patient to bedpan, beside commode, or commode.	___	___	_____
19. Provided for hygiene and assisted patient to bed or chair.	___	___	_____

	S	U	Comments

20. Reinserted rectal tube later if needed or as prescribed.

21. Disposed of equipment.

22. Removed gloves and washed hands.

23. Documented.

Performance Checklist
Skill 31–4

ADMINISTERING AN ENEMA

		S	U	Comments
1.	Obtained equipment.	___	___	_____
2.	Referred to medical record, care plan, or Kardex for special interventions.	___	___	_____
3.	Introduced self.	___	___	_____
4.	Identified patient by identification band.	___	___	_____
5.	Explained procedure to patient.	___	___	_____
6.	Washed hands and donned clean gloves.	___	___	_____
7.	Prepared patient for intervention.	___	___	_____
8.	Raised bed to comfortable working level.	___	___	_____
9.	Arranged for patient privacy.	___	___	_____
10.	Placed waterproof pad under patient's buttocks.	___	___	_____
11.	Placed patient in Sims' side-lying position.	___	___	_____
12.	Arranged top linen and patient gown out of way yet providing privacy.	___	___	_____
13.	Continued procedure according to supplies being used.	___	___	_____

Cleansing enema

		S	U	Comments
14.	Clamped enema tubing 7 inches (28 cm) from end of tubing.	___	___	_____
15.	Filled enema container with appropriately warmed solution and additive required.	___	___	_____
16.	Read disposable package instructions.	___	___	_____
17.	Released tubing clamp, allowing solution to flow through tubing to clear tubing of air; reclamped tubing.	___	___	_____
18.	Hung enema container on intravenous pole so that bottom of container is 12 to 18 inches (30 to 45 cm) above level of patient's anus.	___	___	_____
19.	Lubricated 4 inches (10 cm) of end of tubing.	___	___	_____

	S	**U**	**Comments**

20. Spread cheek of patient's buttock with nondominant hand.

____ ____ _____

21. While rotating enema tubing, gently inserted it 3 to 4 inches (7 to 10 cm).

____ ____ _____

22. Released tubing clamp and allowed solution to flow slowly while holding tube.

____ ____ _____

23. Lowered enema container or clamped tubing if patient complained of cramping and encouraged slow, deep breathing with mouth open.

____ ____ _____

24. Clamped and removed enema tubing when all or enough solution had been administered and encouraged patient to retain solution at least 5 minutes.

____ ____ _____

Commercially prepared enema

25. Removed cover from tip of enema and inserted entire tip into rectum.

____ ____ _____

26. Squeezed container until it could no longer introduce solution.

____ ____ _____

27. Encouraged patient to retain solution.

____ ____ _____

For both forms of enemas

28. When patient could no longer retain solution or all solution had been introduced, assisted to bedpan, beside commode, or commode; reminded patient not to flush commode.

____ ____ _____

29. Provided patient hygiene.

____ ____ _____

30. Assisted patient back to be.

____ ____ _____

31. Disposed of equipment.

____ ____ _____

32. Removed gloves and washed hands.

____ ____ _____

33. Documented.

____ ____ _____

Performance Checklist
Skill 32–1

CARING FOR A COLOSTOMY OR AN ILEOSTOMY

		S	U	Comments
1.	Obtained equipment.	___	___	_____
2.	Referred to medical record, care plan, or Kardex for special interventions.	___	___	_____
3.	Introduced self.	___	___	_____
4.	Identified patient by identification band.	___	___	_____
5.	Explained procedure to patient.	___	___	_____
6.	Washed hands and donned clean gloves.	___	___	_____
7.	Prepared patient for intervention.	___	___	_____
8.	Raised bed to comfortable working level.	___	___	_____
9.	Arranged for patient privacy.	___	___	_____
10.	Inspected adherence and type of pouch.	___	___	_____
11.	Assessed stoma for color, size, and shape.	___	___	_____
12.	Examined peristomal skin for signs of irritation.	___	___	_____
13.	Assessed stool for color, odor, amount, consistency, and frequency.	___	___	_____
14.	Inspected, auscultated, percussed, and palpated abdomen.	___	___	_____
15.	Asked patient whether there were any concerns or discomforts.	___	___	_____
16.	Assessed ability of patient or significant other to perform ostomy care.	___	___	_____
17.	Positioned patient for access to stoma and for patient comfort.	___	___	_____
18.	Unfastened and removed belt (if in use).	___	___	_____
19.	Carefully pushed skin away from pouch.	___	___	_____
20.	Placed reusable pouch on clean area and disposable pouch in plastic bag.	___	___	_____
21.	Cleansed stoma and peristomal skin gently with warm water and gently patted dry.	___	___	_____

	S	U	Comments

22. Applied skin prep to peristomal skin and allowed to dry.

_____ _____ _____

23. Measured stoma using measuring card or custom-made pattern.

_____ _____ _____

24. Placed toilet tissue over stoma.

_____ _____ _____

25. Using pattern or measuring guide, cut opening in pouch skin barrier $1/8$ inch larger than measurement.

_____ _____ _____

26. Removed tissue from stoma.

_____ _____ _____

27. Removed paper cover from pouch skin barrier, centered pouch with skin barrier or flange with skin barrier over stoma, and pressed gently but firmly to skin.

_____ _____ _____

28. Snapped pouch to flange if using two-piece system; attached pouch clamp to bottom of pouch for both one-piece and two-piece pouches.

_____ _____ _____

29. Attached belt if used.

_____ _____ _____

30. Assisted patient to comfortable position in bed or chair.

_____ _____ _____

31. Removed equipment from bedside.

_____ _____ _____

32. Emptied, washed, rinsed, and dried reusable pouch.

_____ _____ _____

33. Disposed of soiled supplies

_____ _____ _____

34. Removed gloves and washed hands.

_____ _____ _____

35. Documented.

_____ _____ _____

**Performance Checklist
Skill 32–2**

PERFORMING COLOSTOMY IRRIGATION

	S	U	Comments
1. Obtained equipment.	___	___	_____
2. Referred to medical record, care plan, or Kardex for special interventions.	___	___	_____
3. Introduced self.	___	___	_____
4. Identified patient by identification band.	___	___	_____
5. Explained procedure to patient.	___	___	_____
6. Washed hands and donned clean gloves.	___	___	_____
7. Prepared patient for intervention.	___	___	_____
8. Raised bed to comfortable working level.	___	___	_____
9. Arranged for patient privacy.	___	___	_____
10. Assessed ability of patient or significant other to perform irrigation.	___	___	_____
11. Positioned patient.	___	___	_____
12. Removed pouch or patch; cleansed skin.	___	___	_____
13. Placed irrigation sleeve over stoma and attached belt if appropriate.	___	___	_____
14. Placed end of sleeve in commode.	___	___	_____
15. Closed clamp in irrigating tubing and filled irrigation container with 500 to 1000 ml of tepid water or as prescribed.	___	___	_____
16. Hung tubing on intravenous pole so that bottom of container was at level of patient's shoulder.	___	___	_____
17. Holding end of tubing over commode, allowed small amount of water to flow through tubing to remove air.	___	___	_____
18. Attached cone to tubing and lubricated cone.	___	___	_____
19. Inserted cone into stoma through top of sleeve.	___	___	_____

	S	**U**	**Comments**

20. While holding cone in place, allowed solution to flow slowly into colon. If patient complained of cramping, slowed or stopped flow without removing cone until cramps subsided. _____ _____ _____

21. After all solution had been introduced, removed cone and closed top of sleeve. _____ _____ _____

22. Had patient sit about 15 minutes while return flowed into commode. Cleansed and clamped bottom of sleeve so that patient could move around freely until drainage stopped. _____ _____ _____

23. Drained, rinsed, and removed sleeve. _____ _____ _____

24. Assessed patient and fecal return and flushed commode. _____ _____ _____

25. Applied new pouch or patch. _____ _____ _____

26. Disposed of equipment. _____ _____ _____

27. Removed gloves and washed hands. _____ _____ _____

28. Documented. _____ _____ _____

**Performance Checklist
Skill 32–3**

CARING FOR A URETEROSTOMY

	S	U	Comments
1. Obtained equipment.	____	____	_____
2. Referred to medical record, care plan, or Kardex for special interventions.	____	____	_____
3. Introduced self.	____	____	_____
4. Identified patient by identification band.	____	____	_____
5. Explained procedure to patient.	____	____	_____
6. Washed hands and donned clean gloves.	____	____	_____
7. Prepared patient for intervention.	____	____	_____
8. Raised bed to comfortable working level.	____	____	_____
9. Arranged for patient privacy.	____	____	_____
10. Positioned patient so that stoma was easily accessible and patient was comfortable.	____	____	_____
11. Emptied urine into graduated pitcher and unfastened and removed belt if in use.	____	____	_____
12. Carefully peeled pouch from skin; moistened cotton balls may be needed.	____	____	_____
13. Covered stoma with rolled gauze.	____	____	_____
14. Placed pouch in plastic bag.	____	____	_____
15. Cleansed patient's skin with warm water and patted skin dry.	____	____	_____
16. Measured stoma using measurement card.	____	____	_____
17. If using wafer-type barrier, cut an opening hole 1/8 inch larger than stoma.	____	____	_____
18. Assessed that skin was free from urine; removed backing from barrier protectant and gauze from stoma. Centered opening hole over stoma and pressed against skin for 1 to 2 minutes, smoothing outward with fingers to remove air bubbles.	____	____	_____

	S	**U**	**Comments**

19. Attached belt to one end of pouch, adjusted around waist, and attached to opposite end. ____ ____ _____

20. Assisted patient to comfortable position in chair. ____ ____ _____

21. Disposed of equipment. ____ ____ _____

22. Washed and dried reusable pouch. ____ ____ _____

23. Measured and assessed urine. ____ ____ _____

24. Removed gloves and washed hands. ____ ____ _____

25. Documented. ____ ____ _____